The Old Age Psychiatry Handbook

The Old Age Psychiatry Handbook

A practical guide

Joanne Rodda
University College London

Niall Boyce
University College London

Zuzana Walker
University College London

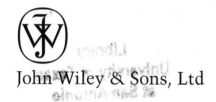

John Wiley & Sons, Ltd

Other Wiley Editorial Offices

John Wiley & Sons Inc., 111 River Street, Hoboken, NJ 07030, USA

Jossey-Bass, 989 Market Street, San Francisco, CA 94103-1741, USA

Wiley-VCH Verlag GmbH, Boschstr. 12, D-69469 Weinheim, Germany

John Wiley & Sons Australia Ltd, 33 Park Road, Milton, Queensland 4064, Australia

John Wiley & Sons (Asia) Pte Ltd, 2 Clementi Loop #02-01, Jin Xing Distripark, Singapore 129809

John Wiley & Sons Canada Ltd, 6045 Freemont Blvd, Mississauga, Ontario, L5R 4J3, Canada

Wiley also publishes its books in a variety of electronic formats. Some content that appears in print may not be
available in electronic books.

British Library Cataloguing in Publication Data

A catalogue record for this book is available from the British Library

ISBN 9780470060155

Typeset in 10.5/13pt Bembo by Aptara Inc., New Delhi, India
Printed and bound in Great Britain by Antony Rowe Ltd., Chippenham, Wilts
This book is printed on acid-free paper responsibly manufactured from sustainable forestry
in which at least two trees are planted for each one used for paper production.

Dedicated to our families, particularly
Linda and Derek Rodda,
and
George and Kathleen Boyce,
and
Rodney and Juliet Walker.

Contents

Preface

Old Age Psychiatry is a growing specialty, due to the expanding proportion of the elderly population, the increasing base of knowledge in this area, and the promise of new diagnostic and therapeutic tools that come with an established and vibrant research community.

The majority of psychiatric trainees will spend some time working in old age psychiatry. All General Practitioners will be confronted with the unique management issues arising from psychiatric pathology in elderly patients. Community Mental Health Teams comprise a number of different professionals, each involved in a different aspect of care but working towards a common goal. This book provides a comprehensive but concise overview of psychiatric, medical and practical issues that may arise within the speciality.

In writing this book, we have been guided by the principle of holistic care. Providing the best care for patients involves understanding and addressing their physical and emotional needs from the point of view of the whole individual including their life story, environment, family and friends. This is the challenge, and the privilege, of treating elderly patients.

Note on the text

Where it may break the flow of the chapter, some information (for example tables and assessment scales) has been included in the form of appendices. The aim of this book is to be a concise guide to Old Age Psychiatry rather than a reference text, and as such suggestions for further reading rather than extensive references are given at the end of each chapter.

Joanne Rodda
Niall Boyce
Zuzana Walker

Acknowledgements

We would like to thank our friends and colleagues for their considerable contributions towards the writing of this book: Dr Darren Cutinha (who helped edit all chapters), Dr Charlotte Boyce, Dr Janet Carter, Dr Claudia Cooper, Professor Gill Livingston, Dr Kallur Suresh, Dr Janet Carter, Dr Rodney Walker and Dr Nick White.

There are many people we would like to thank for their advice, support and encouragement, particularly: Sarah Croot, Lisa Debell, Thomas Dannhauser, Matt Evans and Paul Robinson, Andres Fonseca, Robin Ganz, Maria and Peter James, Amy Lartey, Sara McNally, Shirlony Morgan, Katie and Eoin O'Brien, Yamna Satgunasingam and Tim Stevens.

1

The Assessment of Patients in Old Age Psychiatry

Introduction

Assessment of patients in old age psychiatry follows similar principles to that in general psychiatry, the main differences being in the practicalities and emphasis. Multidisciplinary working is central to the process; in many cases the assessment involves a number of professionals and occurs over a period of time.

The Old Age Psychiatry Handbook   Joanne Rodda, Niall Boyce, and Zuzana Walker
© 2008 John Wiley & Sons, Ltd

Referrals

In general, referrals are made to the appropriate Community Mental Health Team (CMHT, see page 222) and the most appropriate action is discussed in a multidisciplinary meeting. Depending on the nature of the referral, the initial assessment may be completed by one or more members of the team, with involvement of other professionals as necessary.

Beginning the assessment

There are a number of things that it is important to establish at the beginning of the assessment which may seem obvious but make things go a lot more smoothly:

- Introduce yourself and make your role clear – some patients may not realise that they have been referred to a psychiatrist.

- Try your best to put the patient at ease (see above).

- Establish what the patient would like to be called (it's usually best to use Mr/Mrs/Miss if unsure).

- Make sure you know the names of people accompanying the patient and their relationship/roles.

- Ask if the patient would like some time alone without relatives/carers listening (it may be easier to ask at the end, or give the patient the opportunity during the physical examination).

Setting

Assessments usually take place in the patient's home or in the outpatient clinic, although sometimes it is necessary to assess a patient on a hospital ward.

Domiciliary visits

The patient's own home is the ideal environment for an assessment, and allows for a more accurate insight into their social situation and level of functioning, for example:

- Is the house clean, well organised?

- Is there fresh food in the fridge?

- Can they make a cup of tea?

- Can they recognise people in photos around their home?

- Is the accommodation safe/appropriate? (For example heating, hot water, stairs, bathrooms, hazards.)

- Are there empty bottles of alcohol?

- Are there boxes of unused medication?

- How much support is available from people living nearby?

Another advantage of a home visit is that friends and family involved in the patient's care are more likely to be able to attend and give valuable collateral history. This is balanced against the disadvantages of the time necessary for travel, difficulties in performing a physical examination and safety implications for staff. Although the patient may not pose a risk, their environment or other people in the home might. Box 1.1 summarises some important safety and practical procedures.

Box 1.1   Important safety and practical procedures for domiciliary visits

Let the patient and their family/carers know when to expect you.

Plan your route in advance and carry a map.

Familiarise yourself with any history of risk that is available.

Make sure someone knows details of the visit and when to expect your return.

Carry a mobile phone.

If you feel threatened, leave immediately.

Outpatient clinics

The outpatient clinic is the most convenient setting for assessment from the point of view of medical staff, although there are a number of disadvantages:

- It can be disorientating for the patient to travel, which may lead to a less accurate picture of their mental state and cognitive function.

- Friends and relatives are less likely to be able to attend.

- Patients often do not have transport.

Psychiatric wards

It may be necessary for a patient to be admitted to a psychiatric ward for assessment because:

- The patient is at risk of self-harm, self-neglect or harm to others.

- A longer period of assessment is needed than a brief interview at home or in the clinic.

- Family/carers are not able to manage/cope with the patient.

The disadvantage is that the patient is out of their home environment and so the assessment may still not reflect the true level of functioning. In addition, patients might lose some of their skills and confidence.

General hospital wards

Medical and surgical inpatients with acute mental health problems may be referred for liaison assessments on the ward. Before the assessment, read the referral thoroughly and if necessary call the referrer for further information, including any test results pending. It is always worth checking whether or not the patient is already known to psychiatric services, and tracking down the notes if they are.

There are a number of things that you can do to make the liaison assessment go more smoothly:

- Get as much information as you can from the ward nurses.

- Try and arrange for a relative or carer to be present.

- Wards are noisy – find a quiet room where you won't be interrupted.

- Be prepared to do your own physical examination if you feel it is necessary.

- Ask the patient's permission to phone relatives for further collateral information if you need it.

- Be prepared to make more than one visit.

In the case of a liaison assessment the psychiatrist is only *advising* the team looking after the patient of the most appropriate management from a psychiatric point of view. Ultimately, decisions regarding management remain the responsibility of the team looking after the patient.

The psychiatric history in older patients

The psychiatric history follows the same scheme as that used in general psychiatry. There needs to be a greater focus on particular aspects, for example social history and assessment of cognition. In addition, much of the history is often obtained from a relative or carer (see page 10). Box 1.2 gives an outline.

Box 1.2   Overview of the psychiatric history

Source and details of referral

Presenting complaints

History of presenting complaint

  – nature, onset, duration, precipitating factors, impact, risks

Personal history

  – birth and milestones, childhood, education, employment, relationships

Family history

Past psychiatric history

Social history

  – accommodation, finances, activities of daily living, level of support

Past medical history

Medication and allergies

  – note potential interactions and side effects

Alcohol and drugs

Forensic history

Premorbid personality

Collateral history

History of presenting complaint

As with any psychiatric interview, it's good to start with an open question ("can you tell me a bit about what's been happening lately?").

More focused questions can be used to direct the history and to establish:

- Nature of the problem

- Speed of onset

- Duration

- Possible precipitating factors (e.g. life events, physical illness, medication changes)

- Impact on the patient's life (e.g. no longer leaves the house)

- The patient's perception of the problem

- Whether others think there is a problem

- Risks (Table 1.1).

To establish a timeline it can be helpful to relate the onset and changes of symptoms to events like birthdays, Christmas or holidays.

Whilst the patient needs to be able to tell their own story, there are some features that should be screened for, with more detailed questioning where necessary. The nature and range of symptoms experienced by older patients may be different from their younger counterparts.

Table 1.1 Areas of risk to explore in the psychiatric history

Risk to self	Risk to others
Wandering	Aggression
Poor judgement	Disinhibited behaviour
Gas/water taps left on	Poor driving
Poor driving	Gas left on
Self-neglect	
Vulnerability to abuse/exploitation	
Self-harm/suicidal ideation	

Personal history

- Birth and milestones

- Upbringing and significant childhood experiences

- School, higher education and occupational achievements

  - contributes to overall picture

  - gives an idea regarding the patient's previous level of functioning.

- Relationships, marriage and children

- Life events

- Social network.

Many of the current older generation were affected by the Second World War and may have experienced significant adversity. Separation from carers, interruption of education, loss of parents or a spouse and serving in combat with resulting injuries and psychological traumas are all issues that may affect the presentation of psychiatric illness.

It is always important to put life events in to context, for example being a single mother is generally socially accepted in the UK today, but in the past often had devastating consequences.

Family history

Patients with cognitive impairment might seem muddled about the exact names and relationships of family members, and this in itself is informative. Whether from the patient or a carer, it is helpful to obtain accurate information regarding any family history of medical and psychiatric problems.

Past psychiatric history

Patients often use terms like "nervous breakdown" to describe episodes of mental illness in the past. They might also describe diagnoses such as "schizophrenia" which seem questionable. It is often best to ask a few questions about the exact nature of the illness and its treatment to get a clearer picture.

Social history

Interventions aimed at optimising the social situation are often extremely effective and well received by the patient and their family. The main areas to cover in the social history are:

Accommodation

- Type (independent/warden controlled/residential home/nursing home)

- House or flat?

- Rented or owned? (If rented, private or local authority/housing cooperative?)

- Stairs – are the bedrooms/bathrooms upstairs or down?

- Heating (open fires, gas heaters).

Finances

- Are there financial worries or concerns about exploitation?

- Do they receive any state benefits, for example, in the UK, Attendance Allowance (AA), or Disability Living Allowance (DLA)?

- Do they have insight into their financial situation?

- Who controls the finances and is this a formalised arrangement (e.g. power of attorney)?

Activities of daily living

- Is assistance required and how much?

- Personal hygiene

- Dressing

- Cooking

- Eating/drinking

- Shopping

- Use of transport

- Hobbies and interests (past and present).

Current level of support

- Input may be from family, friends, neighbours or paid carers (social services or private). How often do they visit and for how long? What do they do?

- Meals on wheels

- Day centres

- Respite.

Past medical history

Ask about any past illness or surgery, as well as current or chronic conditions and cardiovascular risk factors. These may help with diagnosis or may be exacerbating factors.

Medication

- If the patient doesn't bring a list, call the GP surgery.

- The elderly are particularly susceptible to side effects (see Chapter 10).

- Confusion, anxiety, affective disturbance, psychotic symptoms and falls can all be caused or exacerbated by drugs.

   Ask about compliance, and whether or not the patient has a dosette box or prompting/ help from a carer to take medication. This is also a good time to ask about allergies.

Drugs and alcohol

Ask about past and present alcohol consumption and smoking. Recent changes may reflect the underlying mental state. Drug abuse may not be thought of as a major problem in elderly patients, but is worth asking about.

Forensic history

Ask about any experience the patient has had of the criminal justice system. Recent arrests, convictions and cautions may be important evidence of new-onset psychiatric illness, or a relapse of manic or schizophrenic illness.

Premorbid personality

Premorbid personality is often neglected but can be especially important, for example in the case of disinhibition in frontotemporal dementia.

Collateral History

The law allows us to take information regarding a patient from anyone who wishes to offer it but it is always best to ask the patient for his or her permission. Explicit permission from the patient is essential if you are going to give details of their illness to their relatives. If the patient lacks capacity to give their consent then information can be given to relatives/carers if it is in the patient's best interests. If you are at all unsure, it is best to discuss the issue with a senior colleague.

Ideally, you will be able to take the collateral history in the presence of the patient, allowing the process to be completely transparent. However, it can often be useful to see the patient's relative alone. For example, the relative may wish to discuss behaviour that is upsetting or embarrassing for the patient.

The Mental State Examination (MSE)

The psychiatric history records the symptoms since the onset of illness, whereas the MSE is a snapshot of these symptoms and signs at the time of the interview. In practice, there is considerable overlap between the two. Box 1.3 gives a skeleton plan of the MSE and a more detailed summary is given below.

Box 1.3　Mental State Examination

Appearance and behaviour

Speech

Mood

Thought

Perception

Cognition

Insight

Appearance and behaviour

Awareness

- A reduced level of awareness might reflect effects of physical illness or drugs.

- Rapid fluctuations suggest an acute confusional state.

- Variations in the level of consciousness can also occur in dementia with Lewy bodies.

- The level of awareness will affect performance on cognitive testing.

Appearance

- Personal hygiene: an unkempt appearance and poor personal hygiene suggests personal neglect, although a person might appear well kempt because they are well looked after by a carer.

- Clothing: the state of dress might suggest mania, disinhibition or dressing dyspraxia.

- Environment: on a domiciliary visit the state of the patient's environment also gives clues (cleanliness, tidiness, empty bottles etc.).

Behaviour

- Eye contact

- Facial expression

- Ability to establish rapport

- Anxiety/agitation/aggression

- General slowing/psychomotor retardation/posture

  − can be suggestive of depression, can also occur in dementia

- Overfamiliarity and disinhibition

  − may be suggestive of mania or frontal lobe problems

- Apparent responses to hallucinations

- Tics, mannerisms and stereotypies, for example:

  − as a feature of schizophrenia

  − hyperorality and repetitive behaviours may occur in frontotemporal and other types of dementia.

Speech

- Rate and quantity, for example:

  − ⇓ in depression; can be to the point of appearing to have dysphasia

  − ⇑ in mania, although this is not always the case in the elderly

  − ⇓ may be due to dysphasia (see below)

  − pressure of speech and poverty of speech may reflect mania or depression respectively.

- Tone: may be normal or monotonous (e.g. depression, Parkinson's disease).

- Volume, for example:

− ⇑ in deafness, disinhibition and mania

− ⇓ in anxiety, depression.

- Word finding difficulties:

  − dysphasia (impairment of language, note: this is different from impairment of artic-ulation of speech which is called dysarthria and is due to poor muscle coordination)

  − language deficits are common in many dementias (e.g. semantic dementia)

  − nominal dysphasia (word finding difficulties) occurs early in Alzheimer's disease.

Mood

Depression

The current generation of older people may find it difficult to describe their mood. Biological features and somatisation may therefore be more apparent than the psycho-logical features of depression. The assessment of mood also draws from the assessment of behaviour and both subjective (the patient's) and objective (the clinician's) accounts are recorded. Table 1.2 gives a list of depressive features to screen for. The 15-item Geriatric Depression Scale (GDS, Appendix 1) is a brief assessment scale that can be completed in the clinic.

Differentiating depression from dementia or bereavement can be difficult; for further information see the later chapters on dementia and mood disorders.

If there is any suggestion of depressed mood, enquiry about suicidal ideation is essen-tial. Older men are one of the highest risk populations for completed suicide.

Table 1.2 Features of depression to screen for in the MSE

Psychological features	Biological features
Low mood	Disturbed sleep
Reduced concentration	Disturbed appetite (weight loss)
Anhedonia	Reduced energy
Helplessness and hopelessness	Reduced libido
Bleak view of the future	Complaints of physical illness
Guilty feelings	Diurnal mood variation
Suicidal ideation	
Irritability	
Agitation	

Mania

Mania in older people may present with elation in mood, although often the picture is of mixed affect, agitation, irritability and/or aggression.

Anxiety

- Features of anxiety can occur independently or as a feature of most mental illnesses.

- Anxiety is not uncommon in dementia, especially in the early stages.

- Ask about:

  - background anxiety

  - panic attacks

  - exacerbating factors and coping strategies.

Thought

Thought form

Perseveration   A response appropriate to the first stimulus is given, inappropriately, for further stimuli. For example
"What is your name?"
"Peter."
"How old are you?"
"Peter."
etc.

- Almost pathognomonic of organic brain disease.

- A feature of frontal lobe damage.

Circumstantiality

- Gets to the point eventually but via a circuitous route

- Common in dementia.

Flight of ideas

- Skipping from one subject to another unrelated subject with only a superficial connection.

- A characteristic feature of mania.

- In older people it might not be associated with rapid speech and can be missed.

Loosening of associations

- Occurs in psychosis and other conditions, for example mania.

- The links between topics seem illogical, and can vary from tangential to "word salad".

Thought content

Obsessions

- Obsessions are recurrent and persistent thoughts, images or impulses that the patient tries to but is unable to resist.

- May occur in the context of an obsessive disorder.

- Can also be a feature of psychosis, depression or dementia.

Delusions

- Fixed beliefs based on unsound evidence out of keeping with the patient's social and cultural background.

- Delusions can take many forms and may be associated with a psychotic or mood disorder.

- In the early stages of dementia delusions (especially of theft) may be secondary to forgetting.

- Some types of dementia (e.g. dementia with Lewy bodies) are associated with systematised delusions.

Overvalued ideas

- A belief that may not be unreasonable but is pursued to an unreasonable degree by the patient.

- Often associated with personality disorders.

Perception

Hallucinations in any modality can occur in the context of psychosis, dementia or delirium. Of particular relevance in older people is sensory impairment (i.e. visual impairment or deafness):

- Can lead to hallucinations in the absence of psychosis (e.g. Charles Bonnet syndrome)

- Is an important maintaining factor for hallucinations in the presence of psychosis.

Visual hallucinations are common in dementia with Lewy bodies.

Cognition

Information about cognition is obtained simply by observation throughout the interview, for example:

- General level of orientation

- Ability to follow the conversation

- Ability to remember facts and names during the history

- Asking the same questions/repeating statements

- Presence of confabulation.

More objective testing is mandatory, and in the limited time available in the initial assessment (see below) it is realistic to aim to complete:

- The Mini Mental State Examination (MMSE)

- The clock drawing task

- Bedside tests for more specific cognitive functions, where relevant (Appendix 2).

Insight

Insight may be complete, partial or absent. There may be insight into the presence of a mental illness or dementia but not into the need for intervention.

Assessing cognition with limited time

The MMSE

The Mini Mental State Examination (MMSE, Appendix 3) is a basic 30-point test of cognition over a broad range of areas and provides a quick overview of cognitive function. It is a good idea to make sure that well-meaning relatives know not to prompt answers from the patient, who might become distressed if they are finding the questions difficult.

The score on the MMSE (Table 1.3) must be considered in the context of the overall clinical picture. A low score does not in itself indicate a diagnosis of dementia. Similarly, patients with dementia confirmed by more in-depth neuropsychological testing may score relatively highly on the MMSE, even 30/30.

The MMSE does not contain any items that test frontal lobe function. If there is any suspicion of a frontal lobe deficit then a brief test like category fluency or letter fluency can be performed (see Appendix 1).

Drawing a clock face

Drawing a clock face, writing in the numbers correctly and marking on the hands to show ten past eleven, tests a broad range of cognitive skills and has a relatively high sensitivity and specificity for dementia. It is worth asking the patient to complete this task routinely at the end of the MMSE.

Table 1.3 Level of cognitive impairment associated with the MMSE score (those for dementia are the figures used by NICE for Alzheimer's disease). The score must be interpreted in the context of the clinical picture

MMSE Score	Level of cognitive impairment
27–30	Normal range*
27–30	Mild cognitive impairment*
21–26	Mild dementia
10–20	Moderate dementia
Less than 10	Severe dementia

*Performance depends on age, education and premorbid ability

Testing the function of specific lobes

Where it is relevant, the assessment can be refined by brief "bedside" testing of the functions of one or more specific lobes. This is informative but not a substitute for formal neuropsychological testing. Details of these tests are given in Appendix 1.

Assessment of everyday functioning

This can be divided into activities of self-care (Activities of Daily Living, ADL) and more complex activities of everyday life (Instrumental Activity of Daily Living, IADL). An example of a simple scale is the Bristol Activities of Daily Living Scale. A scale can be given to the carer to complete whilst you carry out the physical assessment of the patient.

Physical examination

Ideally, a physical examination is performed for all new patients. This can be difficult in some circumstances and arrangements may need to be made for it to be completed at a later date. The purpose of the physical examination is to identify:

- Reversible causes of psychiatric illness

- Differential diagnoses

- Exacerbating factors

- Factors that may affect prescribing

- Physical impairments that will affect suitability of accommodation

- Unreported physical illness requiring attention.

Investigations

Investigations are aimed at ruling out reversible causes and facilitating diagnosis and are summarised in Tables 1.4 and 1.5.

Table 1.4 Routine investigations in the old age psychiatry assessment

Blood tests	Full blood count
	Urea and electrolytes
	Liver function tests
	ESR
	CRP
	Thyroid function tests
	Vitamin B12
	Folate
	Fasting glucose
	Cholesterol★
Microbiology	VDRL (to exclude neurosyphilis)★
	Urine microscopy, culture and sensitivity
Neuroimaging	CT/MRI brain now routine in dementia in most old age psychiatry services★

★Not included in Royal College of Psychiatrists guidance for routine investigations in dementia

Table 1.5 Investigations guided by the clinical picture

ECG	For example if there is suspicion of vascular dementia/cardiovascular disease or if planning to use cholinesterase inhibitors.
Chest X-ray	For example, on suspicion of chest infection, heart failure or malignancy.
EEG	Some types of dementia have specific EEG changes. Investigation of epilepsy.
PET	Positron emission tomography. Only available in a few specialised centres. Uses radiotracers to produce images of brain activity. Includes measurements of glucose metabolism, receptors, neurotransmitters, abnormal proteins.
SPECT	Single photon emission computed tomography. Similar to PET, lower resolution but cheaper and more accessible. Used increasingly and may become more common in the future. Measures cerebral blood flow, receptors.
Genetic testing	For example, in early onset AD or if there is a strong family history of dementia.
Lumbar puncture	If suspicion of acute/chronic infection, malignancy.
HIV status	If suggested by clinical picture/risk profile.
Brain biopsy	In exceptional cases.

Table 1.6 Example of a standard memory clinic battery of psychometric tests

Test	Description
Mini Mental State Examination (MMSE)	Screening tool covering broad range of cognitive domains
National Adult Reading Test (NART)	Measure of premorbid intellectual functioning
Cambridge Cognitive Examination-R (CAMCOG)	Tests a wide range of cognitive functions, takes 35–45 minutes
Logical Memory Test, Wechsler Memory Scale III	Very sensitive for verbal episodic memory
Benton Controlled Oral Word Association Test (COWAT)	Detects changes in word association fluency
Halstead Trail Making Test (TMT)	Evaluates processing speed, visual scanning ability, letter and number recognition and sequencing
British Picture Vocabulary Scale (BPVS)	Measure of vocabulary, does not require any reading, speaking or writing skills
Coloured Progressive Matrices	Measures non-verbal intelligence

Neuropsychiatric testing and the memory clinic

Some patients will require a more in-depth neuropsychiatric assessment. This can be carried out by a psychologist or in the memory clinic. The memory clinic assessment provides a more comprehensive assessment of functioning in all cognitive domains. Since the 1980s the number of such clinics in the UK has been increasing. They provide a way of identifying and monitoring patients with cognitive impairment, and their response to treatment. They are also central to a great deal of dementia research.

The assessment generally takes $1\frac{1}{2}$ hours and may be repeated six-monthly or yearly, depending on local protocol and clinical need. Patients who are likely to benefit most are those with mild cognitive impairment (see page 55), mild dementia or those who present a diagnostic challenge. There are a great number of psychometric batteries that can be used; an example is given in Table 1.6.

Table 1.6 gives details of a psychometric battery that could make up a standard memory clinic assessment.

Non-cognitive assessment scales in dementia

Table 1.7 gives examples of some of the major scales used to measure non-cognitive features of dementia. There are quite literally hundreds of assessment scales related to

Table 1.7 Non-cognitive assessment scales in dementia

Parameters measured	Scale	Description
Global severity	Clinical Dementia Rating scale (CDR)	Structured interview, six domains on a five-point scale
Global change	Clinician's Global Impression of Change (CGIC)	Very few guidelines, clinicians assessment of change on a seven-point scale
Activities of daily living	Progressive Deterioration Scale (PDS)	29 items, scores from 0–100. Carer rated
Behavioural and psychological features	Neuropsychiatric inventory	Structured interview with carer, 13 domains, scores from 0–120. Takes 10–15 min
Depression	Cornell scale for depression in dementia	Validated for use in dementia
Quality of life	The Cornell-Brown Scale for quality of life in dementia (CBS)	Semi-structured interview based on previous month
Carer burden	Screen for caregiver burden	25-item self-report questionnaire

dementia and old age psychiatry and it is not possible to provide a comprehensive list here. Further reading is suggested at the end of the chapter.

Assessment of carers

The responsibility of caring for an older person with mental illness often falls to the spouse who is elderly themselves, or to their children who must try to balance their own life against caring for an elderly parent. Assessment of the carers' needs forms part of the overall assessment of the patient. Carers looking after patients with mental illness have a high risk of developing depression.

Summary

The assessment in old age psychiatry is rarely complete after one interview. The higher frequency of organic disease and co-morbid illness leads to a greater emphasis being placed on physical examination and investigations. The wider psychosocial needs of the patients and their carers must be investigated and a cohesive multidisciplinary approach is essential. The use of both cognitive and non-cognitive assessment scales allows objective assessment of severity and monitoring of progress and response to treatment. Box 1.4 gives an overall picture of the initial assessment in old age psychiatry.

Box 1.4   Overview of the initial assessment in old age psychiatry

Psychiatric history

Mental state examination

Physical examination

Assessment scales, e.g.:

  – GDS

  – MMSE

Arrange further assessment as necessary:

  – psychometric testing/memory clinic

  – assessment by other professionals

  – investigations

Arrange follow up

Explanation of what is happening to patient and carers

Further reading

Blazer D (2000) Psychiatry and the oldest old *Am J Psychiatry* 157: 1915–1924

Galloway J (2002) Personal safety when visiting patients in the community *Adv Psychiat Treat* 8: 214–222

Levine JM (2003) Elder neglect and abuse. A primer for primary care physicians *Geriatrics* 58: 37–44

2

Dementia

In 2001, it was estimated that there were 24 million people worldwide with dementia. By 2040, this figure will have risen to 80 million. The majority (60%) of people with dementia live in the developing world, where prevalence rates are rising far more steeply than in the developed world. Dementia contributes more to the number of years lived with disability in those over the age of 60 worldwide than stroke, musculoskeletal disorders, cardiovascular disease or malignancy.

Between the ages of 60 and 64, the prevalence of dementia is less than 1% and after this it rises almost exponentially. In the western world 24–33% of those aged over 85 are affected. The most common causes are Alzheimer's disease (AD, 50–60%), vascular

The Old Age Psychiatry Handbook   Joanne Rodda, Niall Boyce, and Zuzana Walker
© 2008 John Wiley & Sons, Ltd

Table 2.1   Causes of dementia and dementia-like syndromes

Primary neurodegenerative brain disease	Alzheimer's disease
	Dementia with Lewy bodies
	Parkinson's disease dementia
	Frontotemporal dementia
	Progressive supranuclear palsy
	Corticobasal degeneration
	Huntington's disease
	Dementia associated with motor neurone disease
	Creutzfeldt-Jakob disease
Vascular	Vascular dementia
	Subdural haematoma (page 258)
Inflammatory and autoimmune	Vasculitis, e.g. SLE
	Sarcoidosis
	Multiple sclerosis
Infective	Neurosyphilis
	New variant Creutzfeldt-Jakob disease
	HIV
	Post-encephalitis
Trauma	Head injury
	Boxer's dementia (repeated brain trauma)
Metabolic/endocrine	Hepatic/renal failure
	Hypoglycaemia
	Hypothyroidism
	Hyper- and hypoparathyroidism
	Cushing's disease
	Addison's disease
	Renal dialysis
	Chronic electrolyte imbalance
	Hepatolenticular degeneration (Wilson's disease)
Vitamin deficiency	Vitamin B12 deficiency
	Folate deficiency
	Thiamine deficiency (Wernicke-Korsakoff syndrome – page 138)
Toxic	Alcohol
	Heavy-metal poisoning
	Carbon monoxide
Neoplastic	Direct/indirect effects of tumour
Other	Depressive pseudodementia (page 61)
	Normal pressure hydrocephalus (page 264)
	Post-radiation
	Post-hypoxia

dementia (20–25 %) and dementia with Lewy bodies (DLB, 10–15 %) although there are many other causes of dementia and dementia-like syndromes (Table 2.1).

Definition and diagnosis of dementia

In dementia there is an acquired global cognitive impairment, which is usually progressive and irreversible and occurs in the presence of clear consciousness. Deterioration in memory is usually the presenting feature, and there are often deficits in multiple cognitive domains. Apraxia, dysphasia and behavioural and personality changes are common. The ICD-10 and DSM- IV diagnostic criteria for dementia are summarised in Boxes 2.1 and 2.2. These criteria have been criticised for being weighted towards Alzheimer's disease and less inclusive of other types of dementia. They also fail to take into account the variability in personal activities, which means that patients with less demanding lifestyles may not fulfil the criteria when they are clearly demented.

Box 2.1   ICD-10 diagnostic criteria for dementia

Objective decline in memory affecting both verbal and non-verbal material.

A decline in other cognitive activities characterised by deterioration in judgement and thinking.

The decline in memory and thinking causes impairment of personal activities of daily living.

Deterioration in emotional control, social behaviour or motivation.

Clear consciousness – awareness of the environment is preserved.

Box 2.2   DSM-IV diagnostic criteria for dementia

Decline in level of functioning leading to impairment sufficient to interfere with work or social life.

Impaired recent and remote memory.

One or more of: Agnosia, aphasia, apraxia, loss of executive functioning.

Absence of delirium.

Table 2.2 Examples of cortical and subcortical dementia

Cortical dementia	Subcortical dementia	Mixed
Alzheimer's disease	Huntington's disease	Vascular dementia (often classified as subcortical)
Frontotemporal dementia	Wilson's disease	
	Progressive supranuclear palsy HIV related dementia	Dementia with Lewy bodies

Table 2.3 Clinical features of cortical and subcortical dementias

Cortical dementia	Subcortical dementia

Early impairment of:
  − memory
  − language
  − calculation
  − visuospatial ability
	Relative sparing of memory and language
	Slowing of thought
	Depressed mood
	Apathy
	Difficulty with complex tasks
	Impaired coordination
	Movement disorder

Cortical and subcortical dementia

Dementias are often divided into cortical and subcortical based on the site of primary pathology (Table 2.2). The clinical features that are said to be associated with cortical and subcortical dementias are summarised in Table 2.3.

In reality this classification is an oversimplification because most types of dementia show both cortical and subcortical pathology and there is considerable overlap of symptoms.

Assessment of a patient with dementia

An account of the assessment of patients in old age psychiatry is given in Chapter 1. Table 2.4 gives a summary of neuroimaging findings in the different types of dementia.

General management of dementia

A multidisciplinary approach is adopted to ensure optimisation of social, psychological and physical care (Table 2.5).

Table 2.4 Investigations in dementia. DLB, dementia with Lewy bodies; CJD, Creutzfeld-Jacob disease; vCJD, variant Creutzfeld-Jacob disease

Dementia type	CT/MRI	SPECT	PET	EEG
Alzheimer's disease	Hippocampal atrophy (MRI) Generalised cerebral atrophy, ventricular enlargement, widened sulci (MRI/CT)	⇓ perfusion of temporal and parietal lobes 40 % ⇓ perfusion of frontal lobes	Hypometabolism in temporal and parietal lobes	Usually abnormal ⇓ alpha waves ⇑ theta and beta waves
Vascular	Variable dependent on pathologies. May be single strategic infarct or multiple cortical lesions If subcortical ischaemic vascular disease – periventricular and deep subcortical lesions and/or lacunae in basal ganglia and other subcortical areas	Patchy lesions	Patchy lesions	May be normal Focal abnormalities
DLB	Generalised cerebral atrophy Comparative sparing of medial temporal lobes (MRI)	Dopamine transporter (DAT) studies have high sensitivity and specificity – ⇓ DAT in putamen ⇓perfusion of temporal, parietal and occipital lobes	Reduced binding to nigrostriatal projections Hypometabolism in temporal, parietal and occipital lobes	Diffuse slowing Focal delta transients in temporal lobes in 50 %
Frontotemporal	May be focal frontal/temporal atrophy, which can be asymmetrical	Frontal hypoperfusion in 80 %	Frontal hypometabolism	Usually normal
Huntington's disease	May be atrophy of frontal lobes and caudate		Hypometabolism in basal ganglia	Low amplitude waves
CJD	70 % high signal intensity in the caudate nucleus and putamen bilaterally on T2-weighted MRI images	Non-specific changes	Non-specific changes	Typical periodic sharp wave complexes
vCJD	>75 % Pulvinar sign – MRI	Non-specific changes	Non-specific changes	Generalised slow wave activity

Table 2.5   General principles of management of dementia

Area of care	Interventions
Functional	Maximise level of independence with washing, dressing, toileting etc. Appropriate environmental modifications Occupational therapy involvement
Social	Appropriate accommodation Social care package Meals on wheels Financial issues Legal issues (lasting power of attorney etc.) Structured activities Day hospital, day centre
Risk	Identify and minimise risk issues
Pharmacological treatment	Of cognitive symptoms Of behavioural and psychological symptoms
Psychological treatment	A number of psychological interventions may be of benefit; these are described in Chapter 12
Carer support	Education Involvement in decision making Psychological support, e.g. carers groups, Alzheimer's society Respite care
Physical health needs	Treatment of co-morbid physical illness Liaison with GP/hospital teams

Behavioural and psychological symptoms of dementia

The behavioural and psychological symptoms of dementia (BPSD Box 2.3) are often perceived as more distressing than the cognitive features by those who care for people with dementia. Symptoms are often exacerbated by intercurrent illness or changes in routine and environment.

In the assessment of BPSD it is important to establish the nature and frequency of the symptoms and in what context they occur. Minor changes in routine or environment may be the cause of symptoms. It is also important to establish why behaviour is reported as a problem. If the patient is not distressed or at risk as a result of the behaviour and is not causing harm to others then intervention may not be justified.

Wherever possible, the management of BPSD is non-pharmacological. Patients may benefit from a variety of interventions (Table 2.6) although evidence for some therapies is limited.

Box 2.3   Behavioural and psychological features of dementia

Agitation

Aggression

Apathy

Mood changes

Repetitive/purposeless behavioural changes

Wandering

Disinhibition

Hyperorality

Faecal smearing

Poor sleep

Anxiety

Hallucinations

Delusions

Pharmacological management of BPSD

There is limited evidence for the benefit of any medication in the management of BPSD, although over 40 % of patients with dementia who live in care institutions are prescribed an antipsychotic drug. When medication is used, the lowest possible doses are prescribed and the need for continued use is regularly reviewed.

Antipsychotics

The use of antipsychotics may provide modest benefit in BPSD but this must be balanced against the risks associated with their use in dementia:

- High frequency of side effects in the elderly.

- Increased risk of stroke (evidence relates mostly to olanzapine and risperidone but is likely to be associated with all antipsychotics).

- May speed up cognitive decline.

Table 2.6   Non-pharmacological intervention in BPSD

Intervention	Comments
Environment	The ideal environment is familiar, safe and calm (including décor). Wandering is not a problem if the environment is safe and secure. Dim lighting at night reduces confusion/falls if nocturnal waking occurs.
Routine	Predictable routine for mealtimes, bedtime etc. helps orientation and maintenance of circadian patterns.
Reality orientation	Regular reminders of time, day, date, location and peoples' roles and names can reduce frustration, anxiety and consequent difficult behaviours.
Behavioural therapy	Identification of antecedents and consequences of a behaviour can enable modification of triggers and reinforcement of desired but not undesired behaviours. Requires consistency and persistence from carers.
Reminiscence therapy	Memories are triggered by photographs, music and other stimuli. Memories from the distant past may be enjoyable and clearer than recent memories. May provide cognitive stimulation and improve well-being.
Validation therapy	Patients with dementia may retreat into an inner world based on feelings because present reality is too painful. Empathising with these feelings can improve understanding and communication and insight into external reality.
Brief psychotherapies	Some evidence for use of cognitive behavioural therapy and interpersonal therapy.
Family therapy	Exploring difficulties caused by BPSD and how they affect family relationships can help find ways to assist carers to cope.
Complementary therapies	Art therapy, music therapy, multisensory stimulation and aromatherapy can enable patients to express themselves in a non-verbal way. Singing may reduce shouting and agitation. Bright-light therapy may reduce sleep disturbance.
Physical exercise	May improve mood, sleep and self-esteem and divert energy from less purposeful activities.

• Severe side effects and increased mortality in dementia with Lewy bodies. Quetiapine may be the best choice if an antipsychotic is absolutely necessary but there have been no randomised controlled trials (RCTs).

There is evidence that haloperidol may be effective in treating aggression, although there is little evidence for the efficacy of one typical antipsychotic over another. Atypical antipsychotics are associated with fewer side effects. Risperidone and olanzapine may be moderately effective but are associated with increased mortality and risk of stroke.

Valproate and carbamazepine

Mood stabilisers are widely used in the treatment of BPSD, although RCTs have demonstrated no benefit from the use of valproate in BPSD. Evidence for carbamazepine is conflicting.

Antidepressants

Citalopram has been shown to improve BPSD but there is little evidence for other antidepressants. Trazodone reportedly has beneficial effects although an RCT showed no improvement.

Cholinesterase inhibitors and memantine

Cholinesterase inhibitors and memantine may improve cognitive as well as behavioural and psychological features of dementia. If treatment with one of these drugs is prescribed for cognitive symptoms, it is sensible to wait to see the effect this has on BPSD before prescribing further medication.

Benzodiazepines

Benzodiazepines should not be used in the long-term management of BPSD because of the risk of tolerance, dependence and falls. Occasional lorazepam (low doses, 0.5 mg) in the short-term may be helpful if other options have failed (see NICE guidance below).

NICE guidance for the management of BPSD

The NICE guidance for dementia (November 2006) gives guidance for managing "non-cognitive symptoms and behaviour that challenges". This guidance emphasises the importance of careful assessment and cautious use of medication only where non-pharmacological means have failed (Tables 2.7 and 2.8).

NICE also make recommendations for management of co-morbid depression (Table 2.9).

Why differentiate between the dementias?

Accurate diagnosis is essential if a patient is to receive the best care. The patient, carer and family can then have access to appropriate information regarding prognosis and

Table 2.7 NICE recommendations for management of behaviour that challenges

Non-pharmacological interventions	Assess for possible underlying cause Develop and record individual care plan For agitation, tailor interventions to individual's needs; consider, e.g., aromatherapy, multisensory stimulation, animal-assisted therapy, dance/music therapy, massage
Antipsychotics	Consider only if severe symptoms, due to associated risks Discuss risks and benefits, including cerebrovascular risks Identify target symptoms and review regularly Choose drug based on individual risk-benefit analysis Start at a low dose and titrate upwards Monitor particularly carefully for adverse reactions in DLB

Acetycholinesterase Inhibitor	Consider if there are significant non-cognitive symptoms:
	  −DLB
	  −AD, where antipsychotics have been ineffective or are inappropriate
	Do not use in vascular dementia*

*Except as part of well-constructed clinical trials

Table 2.8 NICE guidance for management of behaviour that challenges requiring urgent treatment

Immediate management is in a safe, low-stimulation environment, away from others
Drugs are used with caution to reduce risk of violence and harm
Use lowest possible doses
Avoid high doses and drug combinations
Always offer oral before parenteral medication
Monitor carefully after administration
If intramuscular (i.m.) route is necessary:

  −use lorazepam, haloperidol or olanzapine, preferably as a single agent*
  −if rapid tranquillisation is required, consider haloperidol and lorazepam in combination. Monitor for extrapyramidal side effects (EPSEs), consider anticholinergic** if distressing
  −do not use diazepam or chlorpromazine

*Never use olanzapine and lorazepam i.m. together, because of additive sedative effects
**Caution − may cause confusion, falls and constipation, avoid if at all possible, monitor for adverse effects if prescribed

Table 2.9 NICE guidance for management of depression in dementia

Psychosocial interventions*	Pharmacological interventions

Cognitive behavioural therapy (possibly involving carers)
Range of tailored interventions, e.g.:
  −reminiscence therapy
  −animal-assisted therapy
  −multisensory stimulation
  −exercise
	Risk benefit analysis
	Follow NICE guidance on depression
	Avoid drugs with anticholinergic effects

*Also apply to co-morbid anxiety

support. In addition, the specific diagnosis may affect further management. For example, a patient with dementia with Lewy bodies who is incorrectly diagnosed with Alzheimer's disease may be prescribed antipsychotic drugs without the level of caution required (see below).

Alzheimer's disease

Alzheimer's disease is the most common cause of dementia, affecting over half a million people in the UK, 15 million people worldwide and accounting for approximately 60% of all dementias. It is slightly more common in women than in men even when the increased life expectancy for women is accounted for.

Diagnosis

Alzheimer's disease usually has a gradual onset and steady progression. Diagnosis is dependent on exclusion of alternative neurological, systemic and psychiatric causes. The diagnostic criteria in ICD-10 and DSM-IV are summarised in Boxes 2.4 and 2.5. NINCDS-ADRDA criteria for Alzheimer's disease (Box 2.6) are also widely used.

Box 2.4 ICD-10 criteria for dementia in Alzheimer's disease

Presence of dementia

Usually insidious onset with slow deterioration

No evidence of alternative systemic or brain disease or other possible cause of dementia

---

Box 2.5 DSM-IV criteria for dementia of the Alzheimer's type

Difficulty learning new information and recalling previously learned information

One or more of: Aphasia, apraxia, agnosia, impaired executive functioning

Impairment of work or social function

Gradual onset, steady decline

Exclusion of alternative systemic, neurological or psychiatric cause

---

Box 2.6   Brief summary of NINCDS-ADRDA criteria for probable Alzheimer's disease

Dementia

Deficits in two or more areas of cognition

Progressive worsening

No disturbance of consciousness

Onset age 40–90

Absence of other aetiological factors

Clinical features

The clinical features of Alzheimer's disease are summarised in Table 2.10.

Course and prognosis

Median survival from diagnosis is six years and the decline in cognition and global functioning is usually gradual. Behavioural disturbance and neuropsychiatric features become more apparent as the disease progresses. Superimposed periods of delirium may occur with physical illness.

Factors associated with a more rapid cognitive decline include:

• Age <65 at onset

• Male

• Severe disease

• Apathy

• Depression

• Possibly use of antipsychotic drugs.

Pathology

The characteristic pathological features of Alzheimer's disease are *amyloid* (neuritic) *plaques* and *neurofibrillary tangles*, predominantly in medial temporal lobe structures and

Table 2.10   Clinical features of Alzheimer's disease

Cognitive features	
Amnesia	An early feature is loss of anterograde episodic memory. Ribot's law states that recent memories are lost before remote memories; in reality this might not be the case.
Aphasia	Initially nominal dysphasia (shown by word-finding difficulties). Later, syntax is impaired and speech is increasingly paraphrasic.
Agnosia	Disturbances in object and face recognition.
Apraxia	Loss of motor skills, e.g. difficulty in making a cup of tea. Dressing apraxia (not due to a motor disorder but due to visuospatial deficit). Difficulty in performing complex tasks including planning, organisation, sequencing and abstraction.

Neuropsychiatric features
Depressive features in over half of cases.
Clear depressive episodes in 10–20 %.
Delusions, often relating to theft.
Visual and/or auditory hallucinations in 10–25 %.

Behavioural and personality changes	
Apathy (25–50 %).	Searching.
Wandering.	Disruption of sleep-wake cycle.
Aggression.	Decline in self-care.
Disinhibition.	Coarsening / shallow affect.
Irritability.	Loss of awareness and normal responsiveness to the environment.

the cerebral cortex. There is also loss of neurones, proliferation of astrocytes and loss of synapses.

Amyloid plaques are extracellular deposits of insoluble protein. Their most important component is β-amyloid, which is sometimes called Aβ or A4. β-amyloid and the genes encoding it are central to current theories of the pathogenesis of Alzheimer's disease.

Neurofibrillary tangles are abnormal intracellular structures composed of abnormally hyperphosphorylated tau protein. Tau protein is a normal intracellular protein that binds to microtubules and is involved in axonal transport and maintenance of the neuronal cytoskeleton. It is not clear whether tau protein hyperphosphorylation and neurofibrillary tangle formation are a cause or an effect of Alzheimer's disease.

Less than 50% of patients diagnosed clinically with Alzheimer's disease have pure Alzheimer's pathology. Many have concomitant vascular or Lewy body pathology.

Neurochemical changes

The most pronounced change is of widespread loss of cortical acetylcholine due to pathological changes in cholinergic basal forebrain nuclei. In the early stages there is

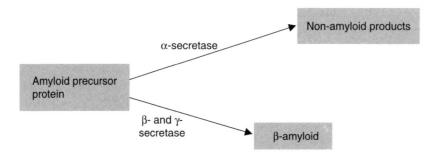

Figure 2.1   Breakdown of amyloid precursor protein

upregulation of choline acetyltransferase. This has led to the development of treatments aimed at correcting the cholinergic deficit.

Aetiology and risk factors

The amyloid cascade hypothesis

β-amyloid is cleaved from a transmembrane protein called amyloid precursor protein (APP). APP is usually broken down into non-β-amyloid peptides by what has been called the α-secretase pathway. The amyloid cascade hypothesis suggests that there is more breakdown of APP by other pathways (called β- and γ-secretase pathways), leading to overproduction of β-amyloid (Figure 2.1).

β-Amyloid is insoluble and is normally cleared from the brain via several different mechanisms. Overproduction results in aggregation and plaque formation.

The relationship between amyloid plaques and tau hyperphosphorylation and tangle formation remains unclear. Many pathogenic mechanisms underlying these changes are under investigation, including inflammation, oxidative stress and cell cycle abnormalities.

Genetic factors

The familial form of Alzheimer's disease is a rare autosomal dominant condition with a prevalence of less than 0.1 %. The majority of mutations are of the presenilin 1 and presenilin 2 genes (part of the γ-secretase complex), and mutations of the APP gene have been found in some families.

There is a significant genetic component to the "sporadic" form of Alzheimer's disease. The majority of the genetic risk can be accounted for by the apolipoprotein E (APOE) $\varepsilon4$ allele, and risk of developing Alzheimer's disease is three times higher in heterozygotes and 15 times higher in homozygotes. APOE $\varepsilon4$ is involved in cholesterol transport in the brain but the exact mechanism by which APOE $\varepsilon4$ predisposes a person to AD remains unclear.

Contribution from other genes has been studied and some suggest that there may in fact be a more heterogeneous genetic basis for the disease.

Risk factors associated with vascular disease

Smoking, hypertension, hypercholesterolaemia, coronary artery disease, obesity and diabetes are all associated with an increased risk of Alzheimer's disease. Smoking alone increases the risk of Alzheimer's disease two- to four-fold.

Cognitive reserve

Individuals with low educational achievement and low levels of physical and mental activity in middle and later life are at increased risk of Alzheimer's disease. This has been linked to the concept of "cognitive reserve". According to this hypothesis, a low cognitive reserve leads to a lower threshold for the disease to become symptomatic.

Head injury

Head injury of any severity is associated with an increased risk of Alzheimer's disease. This risk is increased in APOE ε4 carriers.

Depression

A history of depression is a risk factor for the development of Alzheimer's disease. Depression may also occur secondary to Alzheimer's disease or as a prodromal state.

Down's syndrome

People with Down's syndrome have an extra copy of the APP gene (due to trisomy of chromosome 21) and develop β-amyloid plaques early in life. They have a significantly increased risk of Alzheimer's disease. The risk is also increased in those with a family history of Down's syndrome and in mothers of children with Down's syndrome.

Possible protective factors

Patients and relatives often ask about factors that protect against Alzheimer's disease. Most evidence comes from epidemiological studies and so the differentiation of associations from true protective factors can be difficult.

Table 2.11   Risk factors associated with Alzheimer's disease

Risk factor	Details
Genetic	APOE ε4 Familial (early onset) AD: autosomal dominant inheritance of mutations in presenilin 1, 2 and APP
Risk factors associated with vascular disease	Smoking Hypertension Hypercholesterolaemia Atherosclerosis Coronary artery disease Obesity Diabetes
Brain reserve capacity	Low educational level Reduced mental and physical activity in middle and later life
Brain trauma	Head injury
Other	Depression Ageing

Cognitive reserve

High educational levels and increased physical and cognitive activity in middle/later life reduce the risk of Alzheimer's disease. This protective effect is believed to be due to an increase in cognitive reserve. However, when people with a high cognitive reserve develop Alzheimer's, they may experience a more rapid cognitive decline. These patients may be able to compensate for early deficits by using cognitive strategies, so that the disease becomes apparent at a more advanced stage.

Non steroidal anti-inflammatory drugs

Epidemiological studies have shown that people who take non-steroidal anti-inflammatory drugs (NSAIDs) have reduced risk of developing Alzheimer's. This may relate to the inflammatory properties associated with plaques and has lead to trials of anti-inflammatory drugs in AD. NSAIDS, prednisolone and rofecoxib were found to have little effect when used in treatment of Alzheimer's disease, suggesting that their effect is primarily protective when used in middle and late life.

Antioxidants

There is evidence that Alzheimer's disease is associated with reduced activity of brain antioxidants rendering neurones more susceptible to oxidative damage. A number of substances with antioxidant properties have been investigated, both in terms of disease prevention and treatment. Most evidence is from naturalistic studies but the number of controlled trials is growing.

Vitamin E may protect against Alzheimer's and evidence is stronger for dietary intake rather than supplements. There is evidence for high-dose vitamin E in treatment of AD but also concern about its safety and so it is not routinely prescribed.

Increased intake of fatty fish but not omega-3 fatty acid supplements appears to protect against Alzheimer's. Trials of omega-3 fatty acid supplements in treatment of Alzheimer's disease are ongoing.

Hormone replacement therapy

An association between post-menopausal oestrogen replacement and reduced incidence of Alzheimer's disease has been shown by several epidemiological studies. The relevance of these findings is unclear, as randomised controlled trials show no benefit in prevention or treatment.

Cholesterol lowering drugs

Patients taking statins are less likely to develop dementia, possibly due to reduced amounts of Aβ peptide. Trials of statins in the treatment of Alzheimer's disease have shown no effect.

Box 2.7 Possible protective factors for Alzheimer's disease

High educational level

Physical activity in middle/later life

Mental activity in middle/later life

Antioxidants

Fish oils

Anti-inflammatory agents

Hormone replacement therapy

Cholesterol lowering drugs

Investigations

Investigations in Alzheimer's disease are performed largely to rule out reversible causes of dementia and to help with the differential diagnosis (see page 19). Findings of neuroimaging and EEG studies are shown in Table 2.4.

Drug treatment

Cholinesterase inhibitors

These drugs do not alter the pathology of the disease but increase levels of acetylcholine available at the synapse (see page 198). They improve cognitive function, global outcome and performance in activities of daily living. They may also have an effect on behavioural symptoms. NICE guidelines (Box 2.8) are controversial and seen by many as too restrictive.

Box 2.8   NICE guidance (2006) for cholinesterase inhibitors in Alzheimer's disease

Drugs recommended are donepezil, rivastigmine, galantamine

For moderately severe dementia only (MMSE 10–20)

Treatment may only be initiated by specialists (psychiatrists, neurologists, geriatricians)

Reviews at six-monthly intervals of cognition, behaviour and global functioning

Diagnosis of AD using recognised criteria

Issues of compliance must be considered

Carer's views must be sought

Memantine is not recommended

Cholinesterase inhibitors may be used in patients with an MMSE of >20 but whose level of functioning indicates moderate dementia

Cholinesterase inhibitors may also be used for severe non-cognitive symptoms where non-pharmacological treatment and antipsychotic drugs have been unsuccessful or inappropriate

---

Memantine

Memantine is an NMDA receptor antagonist licensed for use in moderate to severe Alzheimer's disease. It may work by reducing glutamate-mediated excitotoxicity (page 200, Chapter 10). NICE sanction its use only as part of clinical research.

Ginkgo biloba

Extracts of ginkgo biloba (page 201) may produce modest improvements in Alzheimer's disease but evidence is limited and the effect may not be clinically significant. Patients considering ginkgo should be informed that side effects might include gastrointestinal upsets, and that it may increase bleeding risk. Ginkgo inhibits monoamine oxidase and has the potential to interact with other medication.

Vitamin E

A large randomised controlled trial demonstrated some benefit in Alzheimer's disease with high dose vitamin E. The small effect size and concerns about increased mortality mean that it has not become routine practice.

Development of treatments targeted at the disease process

Potential strategies are drugs aimed at:

- Secretase pathways, to reduce production of β-amyloid

- Preventing aggregation of β-amyloid

- Vaccination with β-amyloid or antibodies against it

- Tau and its phosphorylation.

Vascular dementia

Cerebral vascular disease can lead to a spectrum of cognitive changes from mild cognitive impairment to severe dementia. It is the second most common form of dementia, accounting for 20–25 % of cases with onset usually between 60 and 70 years of age. The pattern of impairment varies according to the type and site of pathology; both large and small vessels are important and lead to different clinical presentations. A summary of subtypes of vascular dementia (VaD) is given in Box 2.9.

Box 2.9   Types and causes of vascular cognitive impairment

Post-stroke dementia

Multi-infarct dementia (cortical vascular dementia)

Subcortical ischaemic vascular dementia

Strategic-infarct dementia (single infarct in site where even small loss has dramatic consequences, e.g. thalamus)

Hypoperfusion dementia (secondary to episode(s) of ⇓ blood pressure)

Haemorrhagic dementia (e.g. intracerebral bleed)

Dementia caused by specific arteropathies

Mixed AD and vascular dementia

Vascular mild cognitive impairment

Source: O'Brien *et al.* (2003)

Aetiology

The risk factors for vascular dementia are those for vascular disease in general:

- Hypertension

- Smoking

- Diabetes mellitus

- Hypercholesterolaemia

- Positive family history.

Pathology

Post-stroke dementia

Up to one third of people will develop post-stroke dementia in the year following a cerebrovascular accident (CVA). The underlying pathology is likely to be heterogeneous in nature.

Multi-infarct dementia

Multi-infarct dementia was the classical description of VaD, where multiple large cortical infarcts produce a step-wise decline in cognition. In reality this description applies only to a small number of patients with VaD.

Subcortical ischaemic vascular dementia

Cerebral small vessel disease leads to white matter lesions and lacunar infarcts. The clinical correlates of these two patterns have been referred to as Binswanger's disease and *l'état lacunaire* (lacunar state) respectively but these terms are not particularly helpful. The areas affected are primarily subcortical, including circuitry related to the prefrontal cortex.

Mixed Alzheimer's and vascular dementia

In many cases of dementia post-mortem findings reveal both Alzheimer's and vascular pathology. Both conditions are relatively common and so may occur simultaneously, producing a syndrome of dementia sooner than either would have done alone. There may also be overlap between the two conditions, given that risk factors for VaD are also risk factors for AD.

Clinical features

Clinical features are variable and dependent on the underlying pathology. They may include:

- Abrupt onset or stepwise deterioration – however onset may be insidious and progression gradual with subcortical ischaemic vascular disease

- Fluctuating course

- Focal neurological symptoms or signs

- History of stroke

- Preservation of personality in early stages – however there may be early changes

- Relative preservation of insight

- Depression

- Emotional lability

- Patchy preservation of some cortical functions

- Early impairment of attention and executive function

- Relative sparing of episodic memory compared to AD

Diagnostic criteria

The ICD-10 and DSM-IV diagnostic criteria are shown in Boxes 2.10 and 2.11. ICD-10 further divides vascular dementia into subtypes, including:

- Acute onset

- Multi-infarct

- Subcortical vascular dementia

- Mixed cortical and subcortical vascular dementia.

Box 2.10   ICD-10 diagnostic criteria for vascular dementia

Presence of dementia

Uneven impairment of cognitive function

Clinical evidence of focal brain damage, manifest as at least one of:

  – unilateral spastic weakness of the limbs

  – unilaterally increased tendon reflexes

  – extended plantar response

  – pseudobulbar palsy

Evidence of significant cerebrovascular disease which may be reasonably judged to be aetiologically related to the dementia

---

Box 2.11   DSM-IV criteria for vascular dementia

Impaired memory

At least one of: aphasia, apraxia, agnosia, impaired executive function

Evidence that cerebrovascular disease has caused these deficits, ≥ 1 of:

- radiographic evidence of multiple infarcts of cortex and white matter

- focal neurological signs and symptoms

Symptoms cause material impairment of work or social function and represent decline from previous level of function

Impairments not only present during a delirium

Other diagnostic criteria

The NINCDS-AIREN (Box 2.12) and ADDTC criteria both differentiate between possible and probable VaD. The Hachinski ischaemic rating system (Table 2.12) has been widely used in diagnosis of VaD but is unreliable in differentiating vascular from Alzheimer's dementia.

Box 2.12   Brief summary of NINCDS-AIREN criteria for probable vascular dementia

Dementia

Presence of cerebrovascular disease confirmed by:

- neurological examination

- neuroimaging

Relationship between dementia and cerebrovascular disease supported by ≥ 1 of:

- onset of dementia three months after stroke

- abrupt cognitive decline

- stepwise progression of cognitive deficit

All three of the above must be fulfilled for diagnosis of probable vascular dementia

---

Table 2.12   The modified Hachinski ischaemic
score. Score $\geq$ 5 suggests vascular dementia

Abrupt onset	2
Stepwise deterioration	1
Somatic complaints	1
History or presence of hypertension	1
History of strokes	2
Focal neurological symptoms	2
Focal neurological signs	2
Total	**11**

Course and prognosis

The speed of cognitive decline may be similar to that in AD. Average survival is five
years from onset; approximately 50 % of patients die from ischaemic heart disease.

Investigations

Investigations are as for dementia in general (see Chapter 1). MRI is more helpful than
CT; see Table 2.4. Note that many elderly people may have demonstrable white matter
changes on MRI in the absence of cognitive impairment.

Management

The general principles of management of dementia and of vascular risk factors apply.
In addition, trials have shown limited beneficial effects of cholinesterase inhibitors. This
effect does not seem to be accounted for by co-existing Alzheimer's pathology; enhanced
cholinergic transmission may help to compensate for ischaemic damage to cholinergic
neurones.

Dementia with Lewy bodies

Dementia with Lewy bodies (DLB) was recognised in the 1980s as a subtype of dementia
with distinct clinical and pathological features. It accounts for 10–15 % of dementia cases.

Pathology

Lewy bodies are intracellular neuronal inclusions that stain positive for α-synuclein and
ubiquitin, and are also found in Parkinson's disease. Lewy body disease may form a
spectrum including dementia with Lewy bodies, Parkinson's disease (with or without

Table 2.13 Consensus criteria for diagnosis of DLB

Central feature

Progressive cognitive decline of sufficient magnitude to interfere with normal social or occupational function and:

Core features:	**Supportive features:**
Fluctuating cognition	Repeated falls/syncope
Visual hallucinations	Transient loss of consciousness
Spontaneous motor features of	Severe autonomic dysfunction
Parkinsonism	Systematised delusions
	Hallucinations in other modalities
	Depression
	Characteristic imaging and EEG findings (Table 2.4)
Suggestive features:	**Diagnosis less likely if:**
REM sleep behaviour disorder	Cerebrovascular disease
Severe neuroleptic sensitivity	Other physical illness or brain disorder sufficient to
Low dopamine transporter uptake in	account for clinical picture
basal ganglia on PET or SPECT	Onset of Parkinsonism only at severe stage of dementia

Probable DLB: Two or more core features or;
One core feature plus one or more suggestive features
Possible DLB: One core feature or;
No core features, one or more suggestive features

Source: McKeith *et al.* (2006)

associated dementia) and pure autonomic dysfunction. The pattern of distribution of Lewy bodies in the central nervous system varies between these conditions: in DLB, there are widespread cortical Lewy bodies.

Clinical features and diagnosis

DLB is characterised by a dementia accompanied by fluctuations in cognition, visual hallucinations and spontaneous motor features of Parkinsonism. The consensus criteria for diagnosis (McKeith *et al.* 2006) are summarised in Table 2.13 with further details below. DSM-IV and ICD-10 do not give diagnostic criteria for DLB.

Core features

The presence of two or more core features is adequate for a diagnosis of probable DLB, and one core feature is adequate for possible DLB.

Fluctuations in attention and cognition

- Pronounced variations in attention and alertness

- Can occur from minute to minute.

Visual hallucinations

- Typically well-formed and recurrent

- Tend to occur relatively early

- Often of people or animals.

Spontaneous motor features of Parkinsonism

- Many develop this feature some time after initial presentation

- The picture is usually of gait disturbance and bradykinesia rather than tremor.

Suggestive features

- One or more core feature plus one or more suggestive feature = probable DLB

- No core features, one or more suggestive features = possible DLB

- Suggestive features alone are not enough for a diagnosis of probable DLB.

REM sleep behaviour disorder   There is an association of DLB with REM sleep behaviour disorder. In this condition there is loss of normal muscle atonia during REM sleep resulting in the patient's dream behaviour being physically acted out, sometimes resulting in injury. This may occur before the onset of dementia symptoms. Management includes providing a safe sleep environment for the patient and ensuring the safety of the bed partner. Clonazepam 0.5 mg at night may be helpful.

Severe neuroleptic sensitivity   Patients with DLB are often extremely sensitive to antipsychotic (neuroleptic) drugs. They are associated with severe and irreversible extrapyramidal side effects, impairment of consciousness, autonomic instability and increased mortality. These medications must be used with extreme caution in DLB.

Dopamine transporter studies   SPECT studies of the dopamine transporter (FP-CIT SPECT) show decreased uptake in the basal ganglia in DLB. This correlates well with post-mortem diagnosis and is becoming more widely used as a diagnostic tool.

Supportive features

Supportive features are common but have not been shown to have diagnostic significance. Some of theses features, including falls, syncope and transient loss of consciousness, are explained by the autonomic instability that often occurs in DLB. This may be related to Lewy body pathology in the autonomic nervous system.

Cognitive features

The cognitive deficits in DLB show a distinct pattern with impairment of:

- Attention

- Executive function

- Visuospatial ability.

There is relative sparing of episodic memory in comparison to AD.

DLB and Parkinson's disease dementia

DLB occurs as part of a spectrum of disorders associated with Lewy body pathology, which includes Parkinson's disease. Up to 70% of patients with Parkinson's disease develop a dementia that is clinically indistinguishable from that occurring in DLB. The current consensus is that if features of Parkinson's disease predate the onset of dementia by a year or more, the diagnosis is Parkinson's disease dementia. The one-year rule is an arbitrary cut-off with no scientific basis.

Investigations

Specific findings for investigations in DLB are detailed in Table 2.4. Of note, NICE recommend the use of FP-CIT SPECT (see below) to confirm suspected DLB. Chapter 1 details the assessment of dementia.

Management

The cortical cholinergic deficit in DLB is even more profound than in AD and there is convincing evidence for the use of cholinesterase inhibitors. Antipsychotic drugs should be used with extreme caution (see above). Management is otherwise as for any dementia. Antiparkinsonian drugs can be used in small doses to improve motor symptoms.

Frontotemporal dementia

Frontotemporal dementia is the second most common form of early-onset dementia, and the age of onset is typically between 45 and 65 years (range 21–85). Estimates of prevalence vary, but the peak incidence appears to be 9.4 per 100 000 at age 60–69. Men and women are equally affected and there is a family history of FTD in 40–50 % of cases. Tau is seen as central to the pathophysiology of the disease. Sometimes the term frontotemporal lobe degeneration is used instead of FTD. This is further divided into three clinical subtypes – FTD, semantic dementia and non-fluent progressive aphasia, based on the clinical features and distribution of pathological changes.

Clinical features and diagnosis

The consensus guidelines, which were developed from the Lund-Manchester criteria, are outlined in Table 2.14. HMPAO-SPECT and FDG-PET (see below) are recommended by NICE to differentiate FTD from other forms of dementia.

Subtypes of frontotemporal dementia

The term "frontotemporal dementia" subsumes a number of conditions that have been classified separately in the past. A brief glossary is given in Table 2.15.

Management

There is no specific treatment for FTD. Cholinesterase inhibitors have not been shown to be effective. There is limited evidence that selective serotonin reuptake inhibitors (SSRIs) improve behavioural symptoms.

Less common causes of dementia

Dementia in the context of alcohol abuse

Chronic alcohol misuse can lead to a number of syndromes of cognitive impairment. The Wernicke-Korsakoff syndrome is caused by thiamine deficiency, and in the western world is associated with alcohol dependence in 90 % of cases (see page 138 for details).

Table 2.14 Lund–Manchester consensus guidelines for clinical diagnosis of frontotemporal dementia (1994)

Core features	
Insidious onset and gradual progression	
Early decline in social interpersonal conduct	
Early impairment in regulation of personal conduct	
Early emotional blunting	
Early loss of insight	

Supportive features	
Behavioural disorder	Decline in personal hygiene and grooming
	Mental rigidity and inflexibility
	Distractibility and impersistence
	Hyperorality and dietary changes
	Perseverance and stereotyped behaviour
	Utilisation behaviour
Speech and language	Altered speech output: aspontaneity and economy of speech; pressure of speech
	Stereotypy of speech
	Echolalia
	Perseveration
	Mutism
Physical signs	Primitive reflexes
	Incontinence
	Akinesia, rigidity and tremor
	Low and labile blood pressure
Investigations	Neuropsychological testing: significant impairment on frontal lobe tests in the absence of severe amnesia, aphasia or perceptuospatial disorder
	EEG: normal
	Brain imaging: predominant frontal and/or anterior temporal abnormality

Alcoholic dementia is a separate entity from the Wernicke-Korsakoff syndrome (page 138) and has a different underlying pathophysiology, clinical presentation and prognosis.

Alcoholic dementia

Chronic alcohol misuse is associated with cognitive impairment that appears to be related to direct neurotoxic effects. The picture is, however, complicated by possible contributions from nutritional deficiencies, head injuries and repeated episodes of dehydration, hypotension and/or hypoglycaemia.

Table 2.15 Conditions that are included under the umbrella term of frontotemporal dementia

Disorder	Clinical features
Pick's disease	In the past used for a clinical syndrome of aphasia with dementia, gross frontotemporal atrophy (knife-blade atrophy). At present, this term is only used for histopathologically confirmed cases of frontotemporal dementia with Picks bodies and ballooned cells.
Frontotemporal dementia with motor neurone disease (FTD-MND)	A subset of patients with FTD develop motor neurone disease. FTD-MND has substantially shorter survival (three years).
Semantic dementia	Predominant bilateral temporal lobe atrophy. Fluent, grammatically correct but meaningless speech; loss of word meaning; loss of ability to name objects; word substitution; inability to recognise faces, objects or sensory stimuli; preserved visuospatial ability. Relative sparing of short-term memory and motor skills.
Non-fluent progressive aphasia	Left frontotemporal atrophy. Initial decline in speech fluency, problems with word retrieval, preservation of word understanding, agrammatism. Non-verbal communication unimpaired with preservation of memory, personality and other cognitive functions.
Progressive supranuclear palsy	Subcortical pattern of dementia. Pseudobulbar palsy. Supranuclear palsy. Dystonia of head and neck, Parkinsonism.
Other terms used for FTD	Lobar atrophy, frontal lobe degeneration of non-Alzheimer type, frontotemporal dementia with Parkinsonism, progressive subcortical gliosis, dementia lacking distinctive histology.

CT and MRI scans of alcohol-dependent individuals show ventricular enlargement and atrophy of the cerebral cortex. Both the cognitive impairment and changes shown on neuroimaging are partially reversed by abstinence from alcohol in many individuals.

Management of alcoholic dementia is largely supportive and social and the goal is abstinence. It is also important to address co-morbid medical and psychiatric problems as well as any other sequelae of alcohol dependence.

Huntington's disease

Huntington's disease (HD) is an inherited movement disorder that invariably progresses to dementia. The prevalence is around one in 10 000 and onset is typically in middle life.

Aetiology

HD is an autosomal dominant condition with complete penetrance. This means that offspring have a 50% chance of inheriting the mutation, and all of those who do will develop the disease.

The mutation is a trinucleotide repeat of CAG on the short arm of chromosome 4 that codes for a protein called "huntingtin" whose function remains unclear. The number of repeats tends to increase in successive generations, leading to an earlier onset of increasingly severe symptoms.

Pathology

There is atrophy of the caudate nucleus with loss of GABA neurones. There are also changes in the frontal cortex.

Clinical features

The typical triad in HD is of movement disorder, dementia and a positive family history. Psychiatric features may also be prominent. The condition usually progresses over 10–15 years.

Movement disorder

- Choreiform movements are often subtle at first and may be disguised by the patient

- Accompanied by increased tone and presence of primitive reflexes.

Dementia

- There is a "subcortical" pattern of dementia (page 26)

- Frontal lobe symptoms may be prominent (page 18 or Appendix 1)

- Relative preservation of memory until late in the disease.

Psychiatric features

- Occur in 60–70% of patients

- May be the presenting feature

- Anxiety, depression and paranoia are all common

- Aggression and violence may occur as the disease progresses.

Diagnosis

Specific genetic testing is possible both in the presence of disease and for screening purposes. The results of these tests clearly have enormous implications for the patient and their family and so are best conducted by specialist services.

Management

There is no specific management for HD. Antidepressants can be effective in the treatment of depressive symptoms. Antipsychotic drugs are of less help in the presence of psychotic features but can help to suppress choreiform movements to a limited extent. Sulpiride is usually the antipsychotic of choice. Tetrabenezine can be effective in controlling choreiform movements but can cause depression.

Prion disease

Prion disease is rare, despite widespread publicity over the past decade. Prions are proteins whose exact mode of transmission and replication is unclear, and whose proliferation within the central nervous system leads to a spongiform encephalopathy. Prion diseases recognised in humans in the UK are Creutzfeld-Jacob disease (CJD) and variant Creutzfeld-Jacob disease (vCJD) (Table 2.16).

Human Immunodeficiency Virus (HIV)

Dementia in HIV positive patients may be due to:

- Intracerebral infections such as toxoplasmosis

- Direct effects of the HIV virus.

Antipsychotics should be prescribed cautiously as both the effect of the illness and antiretroviral medication render patients particularly sensitive to extrapyramidal side effects. See page 266 for further details.

Table 2.16   Features of Creutzfeld-Jacob disease (CJD) and variant Creutzfeld-Jacob Disease (vCJD)

	CJD	vCJD
Aetiology	80 % sporadic genetic mutations Few autosomal dominant Few iatrogenic (e.g. pituitary-derived growth hormone)	Consumption of beef from cattle with bovine spongiform encephalopathy (BSE)
Incidence	One per million per year	Less than 200 cases in UK to date
Age of onset	50–70 years	Typically 20–30
Features	Widespread neurological features including: – Myoclonus – Cerebellar ataxia – Pyramidal/extrapyramidal signs Rapid deterioration	Anxiety/depression Personality changes Ataxia Myoclonus Progression to dementia
Diagnosis	Characteristic EEG and cerebrospinal fluid (CSF) findings 70 % high signal intensity in the caudate nucleus and putamen bilaterally on T2-weighted MRI images Definite diagnosis requires brain biopsy	>75 % Pulvinar sign – MRI Tonsillar biopsy
Survival	Less than one year	Less than two years

Mild cognitive impairment

In *mild cognitive impairment (MCI)* there is a cognitive impairment that is greater than would be expected for an individual's age and educational level, but that does not interfere significantly with day-to-day functioning. Operational criteria are outlined in Box 2.13. People with MCI are more likely to develop dementia, progression to probable Alzheimer's disease occurs at a rate of 10–20 % per year.

A great deal of attention has been focused on the concept that MCI may represent an early stage in the natural history of dementia. A subtype of MCI called amnestic mild cognitive impairment has been shown to put individuals at high risk of developing Alzheimer's disease. Identification of patients at an early stage of dementia may lead to a better understanding of the underlying processes and provide avenues for research and the development of new interventions.

Box 2.13   Criteria for mild cognitive impairment

Memory complaint, corroborated by an informant

Abnormal memory function (≥ 1.5 SD below age-appropriate norm)

Normal general cognitive function (verbal or performance IQ within 0.5 SD)

No or minimal impairment in activities of daily living

Do not meet criteria for dementia

Source: Petersen *et al.* (1999)

Functional and molecular neuroimaging in dementia

CT and MRI (structural neuroimaging) are widely used in the assessment of dementia, mainly to exclude other pathologies. MRI is preferable, particularly if vascular changes are suspected. More recently, functional and molecular neuroimaging methods are being used to facilitate diagnosis of dementia and as a research tool.

Functional neuroimaging includes studies of regional blood flow, which is tightly coupled with metabolism. Examples are fMRI, HMPAO-SPECT and FDG-PET. *Molecular neuroimaging* techniques rely on binding of ligands to receptors or other specific proteins in the brain and include FP-CIT SPECT. These investigations are outlined below.

Single-photon emission tomography (SPECT)

SPECT uses gamma cameras to detect gamma rays emitted by injected tracers. The most common tracer used in neuroimaging with SPECT is ^{99m}Tc-hexamethylpropylene amine oxime (^{99m}Tc-HMPAO-SPECT). The ^{99m}Tc emits gamma rays that are detected by a gamma camera. When it is attached to HMPAO it is taken up by brain tissue in a manner that it enables measurement of regional blood flow. HMPAO-SPECT can be helpful in differentiating Alzheimer's, frontotemporal and vascular dementias based on the pattern of cortical perfusion deficit.

SPECT is also helpful in diagnosis of DLB, using a radiolabelled ligand (FP-CIT) that binds to presynaptic dopamine transporters. Patients with DLB have markedly reduced of FP-CIT uptake in the striatum.

Positron emission tomography (PET)

In PET, a radioactive tracer isotope is attached to a molecule that is then injected into the subject. It differs from SPECT because the radioisotope undergoes positron emission decay, which ultimately results in the release of two photons moving in opposite directions. These photons are simultaneously detected by a scintillator and used to construct a three-dimensional image.

PET scanning is far less widely available than SPECT, principally because the isotopes used are very short-lived and need to be produced using expensive and highly specialised equipment. The most commonly used radiotracer in PET is [^{18}F]flourodeoxyglucose (FDG). FDG-PET can be used in a similar way to HMPAO-SPECT to differentiate between dementia subtypes.

Functional magnetic resonance imaging (fMRI)

Functional MRI uses the differences in magnetic resonance signal between oxygenated and deoxygenated haemoglobin. It is then possible to measure blood flow to (and therefore activation of) different brain areas during activity, for example performance on tests of a specific cognitive domain. The use of fMRI in research is growing exponentially, and it may one day have a role in early diagnosis and differentiation of dementia.

NICE guidance and neuroimaging in dementia

NICE recommend that MRI or CT is used to exclude other pathology and to help establish the subtype of dementia. They also recommend the use of:

- HMPAO-SPECT (or alternatively FDG-PET) to help differentiate Alzheimer's disease, vascular dementia and frontotemporal dementia

- FP-CIT SPECT to confirm suspected DLB.

Further reading

Blennow K, de Leon MJ and Zetterberg H (2006) Alzheimer's disease *Lancet* 368: 387–403

Douglas S, James I and Ballard C (2004) Non-pharmacological interventions in dementia *Adv Psychiat Treat* 10: 171

Ferri CP, Prince M, Brayne C et al. (2005) Global prevalence of dementia: a Delphi consensus study *Lancet* 366: 2112–2117

Gauthier M, Reisberg B, Zaudig M et al. (2006) Mild cognitive impairment *Lancet* 367: 1262–1270

Grundman M, Petersen RC and Ferris SH et al. (2004) Alzheimer's Disease Cooperative Study. Mild cognitive impairment can be distinguished from Alzheimer disease and normal aging for clinical trials *Arch Neurol* 61: 59–66

Klafki HW, Staufenbiel M, Kornhuber J and Wiltfand J (2006) Therapeutic approaches to Alzheimer's disease *Brain* 129: 2840–2855

Lléo A, Greenberg SM and Growdon JH (2006) Current pharmacotherapy for Alzheimer's disease *Annu Rev Med* 57: 513–533

Lopez OL, Kuller LH and Becker JT (2004) Diagnosis, risk factors and treatment of vascular dementia *Curr Neurol Neurosci Rep* 4: 358–367

McKeith IG (2006) Consensus guidelines for the clinical and pathologic diagnosis of dementia with Lewy bodies (DLB): report of the Consortium on DLB International Workshop *J Alzheimers Dis* 9(3 Suppl): 417–423

Neary D, Snowdon J and Mann D (2005) Frontotemporal dementia *Lancet Neurol* 4: 771–780

O'Brien J, Erkinjuntti T, Reisberg B et al. (2003) Vascular cognitive impairment *Lancet Neurol* 2(2): 89–98

O'Brien J, McKeith I, Ames D and Chiu E (2006) *Dementia with Lewy Bodies and Parkinson's Disease Dementia* London, Taylor and Francis

Schneider LS, Tariot PN, Dagerman KS et al. (2006) CATIE-AD Study Group. Effectiveness of atypical antipsychotic drugs in patients with Alzheimer's disease *N Engl J Med* 355(15): 1525–1538

Petersen RC, Smith GE, Waring SC et al. (1999) Mild cognitive impairment: clinical characterization and outcome *Arch Neurol* 56(3): 303–308.

Sink KM, Holden KF and Yaffe K (2005) Pharmacological treatment of neuropsychiatric symptoms of dementia. A review of the evidence *JAMA* 293: 596–608

3
Depression

Depression is a common problem in the elderly and is often under-recognised and under-treated. The clinical picture may be different from that in younger adults, and there is frequently co-morbid physical illness or dementia. Other age-related physical and psychosocial factors also increase the vulnerability of elderly people to depression. Despite these differences, treatment of depression in the elderly is as effective as in younger adults.

Whilst the majority of cases of depression in old age will be unipolar disorder, bipolar illness may occasionally emerge in old age. This is covered in more detail later in Chapter 4.

Epidemiology

The prevalence of depression in the elderly varies according to the population sampled and the diagnostic criteria used. Based on DSM-IV criteria for major depressive disorder,

The Old Age Psychiatry Handbook   Joanne Rodda, Niall Boyce, and Zuzana Walker
© 2008 John Wiley & Sons, Ltd

Table 3.1 Prevalence of major depression in the elderly in different settings

Location	Prevalence
Community	0.9–9.4 %
Hospitals	10–12 %
Nursing homes	14–42 %

community prevalence is up to 9.4 %. This figure is higher in hospitals and nursing homes (Table 3.1). Both the prevalence and the incidence of major depression double after the age of 70. The male:female ratio is 1:2, although there is evidence that this ratio evens out in the very old.

Clinical features and diagnosis

The diagnostic criteria for depression are summarised in Table 3.2. Diagnosis of depression requires careful assessment and exclusion of other causes; details are given in Chapter 1.

The list of depressive features in DSM-IV is very similar to ICD-10. In DSM-IV five or more symptoms must be present for two weeks for *major depressive disorder*. One of these must be depressed mood or reduced enjoyment. *Minor depressive disorder* is diagnosed if less than five symptoms are present.

In ICD-10 mild and moderate depressive episodes are coded as occurring with or without a *somatic syndrome* (Box 3.1). Somatic features are common in depression in the elderly, and can be helpful diagnostically if patients find it difficult to talk about their mood.

Table 3.2 ICD-10 diagnostic criteria for depression

Core features	Other features
Depressed mood for at least two weeks	Loss of confidence or self-esteem
Anhedonia*	Feelings of guilt
Reduced energy	Suicidal thoughts or behaviour
	Reduced concentration
	Psychomotor agitation or retardation
	Sleep disturbance
	Change in appetite or weight

Mild depressive episode: ≥2 core features, total of 4–5 features overall.

Moderate depressive episode: ≥2 core features, total of 6–7 features overall.

Severe depressive episodes: all 3 core features, at least 5 other features. With or without psychotic features.

*Loss of interest or pleasure in activities that were normally pleasurable

---

Box 3.1   ICD-10 somatic syndrome

Loss of interest in things that are normally pleasurable

Lack of emotional reactions to things that normally produce an emotional response

Early morning waking (>2 hours before normal)

Depression worse in morning

Marked psychomotor retardation or agitation

Loss of appetite

Weight loss (≥5 % in previous month)

Loss of libido

Four symptoms must be present to qualify for somatic syndrome

---

Some depressive symptoms are more common in the elderly and may be the presenting features. These include:

- Anxiety

- Somatic complaints

- Cognitive impairment

- Psychomotor agitation (agitated depression)

- Psychotic symptoms.

Symptoms like apathy, fatigue and reduced appetite may be difficult to differentiate from symptoms of physical illness.

Cognitive impairment in depression

The elderly are particularly susceptible to reversible cognitive impairment during a depressive episode (depressive pseudodementia) and this has been linked to the concept of reduced cognitive reserve. Some will fully recover but many will have persistent deficits on remission. At least 40 % will develop dementia within three years and 70 % within seven years. Depression in dementia is discussed in more detail on page 72.

Elderly people who develop cognitive impairment in depression are less likely to have a family history of depression or a history of depression in younger adult life.

Psychotic features

Psychotic features are more common in depression in the elderly than in younger adults. Delusions are typically of guilt, nihilistic, persecutory or hypochondriacal. Hallucinations can occur in any modality. Delusions and hallucinations are usually mood-congruent.

Dysthymia

In dysthymia low intensity symptoms of depression are present for two years or longer. These patients may appear generally dissatisfied with life but do not meet the criteria for diagnosis of a depressive episode.

Some patients with dysthymia will go on to develop depression, and this is particularly relevant in the very elderly. In this group, a subsyndromal phase of up to three years may precede depression. Estimates of the prevalence of dysthymia in the elderly are in the region of 2 % in the community and 10 % in primary care.

Risk factors for depression in old age

Many risk factors for depression are associated with age although old age in itself is not a risk factor. The most important risk factors for depression in old age are summarised below.

Genetic risk

There is some genetic contribution to depression in late life but this is weaker than in younger adults.

Physical illness

The comparatively high risk of depression in the elderly is largely explained by the prevalence of physical illness. A higher burden of medical problems correlates with an increased incidence of depression in older people.

Any medical illness may be a precipitating factor for depression. Major causes are listed in Box 3.2. Conversely, depression may increase the likelihood of negative outcomes (including mortality) in physical illness.

Cardiovascular disease

Of patients who have had a *myocardial infarction* or who are undergoing angiography 25 % have minor depression, whilst 25 % have major depression. Of those with major depression at the time of cardiac catheterisation 50 % will still be depressed a year later. *Hypertension* has also been associated with depression by some researchers.

Cerebrovascular disease

Depression develops in one third of patients who have survived ischaemic *stroke*. Risk appears to be associated with stroke severity, physical disability and cognitive impairment. Diffuse cerebrovascular changes may also be important in the aetiology of late-life depression, and a vascular subtype of depression has been proposed (see below).

Endocrine disorder

Thyroid and parathyroid disorder, hyper/hypoadrenocorticism and Cushing's disease may all cause a depressive syndrome. The prevalence of depression in *diabetic* patients is approximately 20 %.

Box 3.2   Medical illnesses associated with depression

Infections

Endocrine disorder (thyroid, parathyroid, adrenal cortical disorder)

Malignancy

Diabetes

Myocardial infarction

Cerebrovascular disease

Parkinson's disease

Malnutrition

Vitamin B12 deficiency

Dementia

Other physical illnesses and depression

Depression occurs in 25–38 % of those with *malignancy* and the prevalence of depressive symptoms is approximately 50 % in patients with *Parkinson's disease*. Depression is also associated with metabolic abnormalities including malnutrition and vitamin B12 deficiency. The incidence of depression is also increased in dementia; this is discussed on page 72.

Vascular depression

There is evidence that cerebrovascular disease predisposes to, precipitates or exacerbates depression in late life and a specific syndrome of vascular depression has been suggested. Evidence to support this includes:

- Co-morbidity of depression, cerebrovascular lesions and cerebrovascular risk factors.

- Association between late life depression and MRI changes in deep white matter, periventricular white matter and subcortical grey matter.

- Correlation between both functional impairment in depression and poor response to antidepressant treatment, and white matter changes.

The pattern of clinical features is different from that in non-vascular depression, particularly with respect to cognitive and functional impairment and psychomotor symptoms (Box 3.3). A family history of depression is less likely in patients with vascular depression.

Box 3.3   Clinical features in vascular vs. non-vascular depression in the elderly

Greater disability and cognitive impairment

Pronounced cognitive impairment in terms of verbal fluency and object naming

Prominent symptoms of

  – apathy

  – retardation

  – lack of insight

Relatively lower prevalence of agitation and guilt

There may be advantages to recognition of vascular depression as a distinct clinical entity. For example, management of cardiovascular risk factors may reduce the risk of vascular depression. Some antidepressants are reported to promote ischaemic recovery (e.g. drugs that enhance dopaminergic and noradrenergic action), and may be beneficial in vascular depression. Finally, recognition may be of prognostic value.

Medication

Many drugs are associated with depression. Table 3.3 lists some common examples but is by no means exhaustive.

Psychological risk factors

Cognitive style

Depression in old age has been associated with several cognitive distortions and thinking styles such as rumination, catastrophic thinking, external locus of control and low levels of mastery.

Personality disorder

Avoidant and dependent personality disorders are particularly strongly associated with depression in the elderly. Personality disorders in depressed older patients are predictive of a poorer outcome in terms of persistence and re-emergence of depressive symptoms.

Table 3.3 Drugs that may cause depression

Psychiatric drugs	Benzodiazepines, mood stabilisers
Cardiovascular medication	Antihypertensives – clonidine, methyldopa, beta-blockers, calcium-channel blockers, ACE inhibitors, reserpine. Some evidence for statins
Gastrointestinal drugs	H2 receptor antagonists e.g. cimetidine
Hormones	Oestrogens, progesterone, selective oestrogen-receptor modulators
Oncology medication	Tamoxifen, vinblastine, vincristine
Analgesics	NSAIDs
Others	Steroids Antiparkinsonian drugs Some antibiotics Alcohol and substance misuse

Protective factors

It is possible that changes of attitude in old age reduce the impact of psychological risk factors. For example, the elderly may prioritise "time left" rather than previous experience and thus prioritise positive emotional experiences. The increase in "wisdom" (as defined by researchers) with age may be protective.

Social factors

There are many social stressors in old age that may increase the risk of depression. These include:

- Social isolation

- Low economic and social status

- Relocation

- Impact of disability on independence, relationships and self-image

- Bereavement and other life events.

Bereavement

Up to one third of bereaved elderly spouses will meet the criteria for a depressive episode during the year following the bereavement. Although some see this as a normal response to adversity, these individuals can benefit from treatment of their depression. Responses to grief and depression in the context of bereavement are discussed on pages 73–75.

Table 3.4 Summary of risk factors for late life depression

Biological	Psychological	Social
Genetic	Cognitive impairment	Social isolation
Co-morbid medical illness	Personality disorder	Lower socioeconomic status
Pain	Insomnia	Relocation
Cerebrovascular disease		Disability
		Bereavement

Pathophysiology

Numerous pathophysiological mechanisms have been implicated in late life depression. These include:

- *Serotonergic depletion.* A decline in serotonergic activity occurs between youth and middle age. However, this appears to "level off" in later life.

- *Endocrinological changes*, for example decline in serum testosterone.

- *Abnormalities of frontostriatal circuitry.*

- *Abnormalities of the amygdala and hippocampus*, which may be related to both aging and hypercortisolaemia.

Treatment

In all elderly patients with depression an important part of management is the detection and treatment of underlying physical illness, review of medication and alcohol intake and appropriate involvement of allied healthcare professionals to optimise physical health and function.

In mild depression, "watchful waiting" may be an appropriate strategy, but if symptoms persist for more than two or three months then treatment should be started.

Pharmacological treatment

Antidepressant medication is as effective in the elderly as it is in younger patients. Details about individual classes and drugs are given in Chapter 10, and an outline of the principles of treatment is given below.

Choice of drug

There is no clear evidence that any one antidepressant works better than any other, but the selective serotonin reuptake inhibitors (SSRIs) appear to have the safest side-effect profile and are recommended as first line drugs by NICE. This is supported by the findings of a recent Cochrane review of drug treatment of depression in the elderly. This review also found that tricyclic-related antidepressants (e.g. trazodone) are as safe and effective as SSRIs.

If an SSRI is ineffective or not tolerated, there is little point in switching to another SSRI. A trial of at least six weeks is necessary before changing antidepressant because of inefficacy, because there is often a longer delay in onset of action of antidepressants in the elderly. It is also important to confirm adherence to treatment.

Second line drugs include venlafaxine and mirtazapine. Tricyclic antidepressants and moclobemide are generally used as a third line and side effects must be carefully considered before prescribing.

SSRIs are also the drug of choice in most cases for treating patients with co-morbid medical illness, although there is less agreement about their efficacy.

Patient factors are also taken into account when choosing the most appropriate antidepressant. Some side effects may be unacceptable in certain patients (e.g. risk of gastrointestinal bleeding or osteoporosis with SSRIs). However, side effects like sedation (trazodone and mirtazapine) and weight gain (mirtazapine) may in fact be beneficial for some patients.

Box 3.4   Important information for patients when starting an antidepressant

Delay in onset of action

Side effects

Withdrawal symptoms may occur if stopped suddenly but the tablets are not addictive

Need for maintenance treatment

Other options are available if this treatment is not effective

---

Duration of treatment

There is evidence that older people are more likely to experience relapse when antidepressant medication is stopped. There is no clear consensus, but continuing treatment for at least one to three years after resolution of symptoms may be the best approach. If there are significant risks of relapse (e.g. ongoing social stress, previous relapses), treatment may need to be lifelong. Some advocate lifelong maintenance treatment following any depressive episode in old age.

Augmentation

Patients who do not respond to trials of two or more antidepressant drugs may benefit from augmentation treatment. The strongest evidence for augmentation treatment in the elderly is for lithium, which can be very effective. However, because of the potential side effects and need for monitoring (page 181), this will not be an acceptable or safe option for all patients.

There is very little evidence for other augmentation strategies (e.g. combination of an SSRI and a tricyclic antidepressant) in the elderly.

Management of psychotic features

Psychotic features in depression in the elderly may be less responsive to antipsychotic drugs than in younger adults but there is little evidence to draw on. The likely side effects of antipsychotics need to be balanced against any potential benefits. A generally accepted approach is the use of an SSRI or venlafaxine in combination with an atypical antipsychotic or ECT. Many advocate the use of ECT as first line in these patients.

Psychological treatment

The psychological therapies with the largest evidence base in the elderly are:

• Cognitive behavioural therapy (CBT)

• Problem-solving therapy

• Interpersonal therapy.

CBT, or CBT combined with antidepressant therapy, appears to be more effective than antidepressant treatment alone. There is less evidence for these therapies in those with co-morbid physical illness.

In cases where the patient finds transport difficult or lives in an inaccessible area, minimal contact bibliotherapy, consisting of a literature and telephone-contact based therapy following an initial assessment, may be of use.

When the use of psychological therapies is limited by dementia, behavioural therapy or reminiscence therapy may be beneficial.

Education about depression can also help both the patient and their family to cope with the illness.

Electroconvulsive therapy (ECT)

Electroconvulsive therapy (ECT) is an effective treatment for severe depression in the elderly, particularly when the illness is associated with psychotic features. Indications for ECT in depression include:

• Life-threatening refusal of food or fluid

- High suicide risk

- Failure of antidepressant treatment.

Response rates are reported to be as high as 80–90 % in the elderly, although they are lower if an initial trial of pharmacological treatment has been unsuccessful. There are high relapse rates in the weeks following ECT. To avoid relapse it is therefore essential that antidepressant treatment continues. ECT is covered in more detail on pages 206–212.

Social intervention

Optimising support and social contact at home or moving to more appropriate accommodation can help to remove a great deal of social stress. Social support and contact is also provided by day centres or day hospitals, which can be of benefit in helping the patient to recover from depression, and to build up a social network to protect against future relapse.

There is also evidence to suggest that exercise is of benefit in reducing negative mood symptoms in older patients, including those with medical illness and dementia.

Table 3.5 Summary of the management of depression in the elderly

Pharmacological	SSRI usually first choice
	May take longer before onset of action
	Maintenance treatment often lifelong
Psychological	CBT and medication more effective than either alone
	Other options:
	– problem solving therapy
	– interpersonal therapy
Social	Maximise social support and contact
	Appropriate accommodation
	Day centre/hospital
	Exercise programs
ECT	Severe depression with high risk of suicide
	Poor response to drug treatment
	Life-threatening food/fluid refusal
	Psychotic features
Management of psychotic features	ECT
	Atypical antipsychotics

Outcome

Remission

The treatments that are available for depression are as effective for older adults as they are for younger adults. However, depression is often under-recognised and under-treated in the elderly.

After two years, 21 % of elderly patients with depression will have died, and almost 50 % will still have depression. However, it is difficult to disentangle the confounding effects of physical illness, cognitive impairment, long-term mental illness, social stressors, and different management approaches in elderly patients.

Non-suicide mortality

Depression is associated with increased non-suicide mortality in patients both with and without dementia. It is not known whether this is a result of the effect of physical illness on mental state or vice versa. The effect of treatment of depression on mortality is unclear.

Suicide

Elderly people form the highest risk group for completed suicide worldwide. Furthermore, of those who attempt suicide, the elderly are the most likely to die. Depression is present in up to 83 % of elderly suicides, and is a more common association than in younger adults.

The risk of suicide must not be underestimated in the elderly, and opportunities must be taken to specifically ask about suicidal ideation or plans. This issue is covered in more detail on pages 76–78.

Prevention of depression in the elderly

A number of prevention strategies for depression have been investigated in the elderly. Overall the evidence is limited, but the four brief (12 weeks or less) interventions that appear to have some effect in preventing depression in elderly subjects are:

- Individual therapy for bereaved "at risk" subjects

- Educational interventions for subjects with chronic illness

- CBT interventions targeted at negative thinking

- Life review.

Given the strong links between depression and vascular disease, it has been suggested that management of cardiovascular risk factors might have a protective effect.

Depression and dementia

Symptoms of depression sometimes precede cognitive impairment and dementia in Alzheimer's disease. Those who experience cognitive impairment in depression in old age are likely to develop dementia within a few years of the onset of depression. Depression in early life is also a risk factor for dementia.

The point prevalence of depression in patients with Alzheimer's disease is estimated at 17 %, and is higher in some other types of dementia. Although it is common, diagnosis of depression in dementia can be difficult. The US National Institute of Mental Health (NIMH) has developed provisional criteria for diagnosis of depression in Alzheimer's disease (Box 3.5).

Box 3.5   Provisional NIMH criteria for depression in Alzheimer's disease

$\geq$3 depressive symptoms present in a two-week period

Symptoms representing change from previous functioning

One of these symptoms must be one of:

  −depressed mood

  −decreased positive affect

  −decreased pleasure

Other symptoms may be:

− social isolation or withdrawal	− feelings of worthlessness
− appetite disturbance	− feelings of hopelessness
− sleep disturbance	− excessive or inappropriate guilt
− psychomotor agitation/retardation	− recurrent thoughts of death
− irritability	− suicidal ideation or behaviour
− fatigue or loss of energy	

Symptoms must not be a result of a dementia syndrome (e.g. weight loss secondary to problems with food intake)

Depression must not be caused by other mental or physical illness or medication

---

Depression in dementia is associated with:

- Impaired activities of daily living and more rapid decline in function

- Lower quality of life in general

- Increased probability of physical aggression

- Higher likelihood of transfer to nursing home care.

Management of depression in dementia involves addressing social and psychological factors (see above) as well as medication. Citalopram has been shown to be safe and effective although trials of medication are limited. Cholinesterase inhibitors may also have some effect on depressive symptoms that occur in the context of dementia.

Bereavement

Bereavement refers to the loss through death of a loved one and is an event faced by many in old age. Some interpret the term more broadly to include those who have undergone a recent major life change such as a move from independent living to residential care, or a debilitating illness in a spouse. Bereavement is associated with increased psychiatric and medical morbidity and there is increased mortality from all causes in the six months following the bereavement. "Normal" responses to bereavement can be mistaken for psychiatric illness, and an understanding of the process of grief is important for all healthcare professionals.

Normal grief reaction

By convention, the normal grief reaction is described in several stages (Table 3.6). This approach is helpful, although in practice the process is continuous. Symptoms do not necessarily occur in a specific order and each individual will respond differently to their loss.

Reactivation of symptoms, for example on anniversaries, is common after apparent resolution.

Abnormal (pathological) grief

In *abnormally intense grief*, symptoms are unusually severe and meet the criteria for a depressive episode. Given the nature of the process of normal grief, this can be difficult

Table 3.6 Normal grief

Stage 1 Days ~ two weeks	Numbness Denial Disbelief
Stage 2 Weeks ~ six months	Preoccupation with the deceased Yearning, pining and waves of grief with autonomic symptoms Restlessness Guilt, anger Poor sleep and appetite Illusions, vivid imagery, transient visual hallucinations of deceased Hallucinations of the voice of the deceased Feeling of the deceased being present
Stage 3 Weeks ~ months	Resolution of symptoms Acceptance

to establish. DSM-IV outlines features that are suggestive of depression rather than a normal grief reaction (Box 3.6).

Box 3.6 Features suggestive of depression rather than normal grief (DSM-IV)

Feelings of guilt not related to events surrounding the death of the loved one

Thoughts of death that are not related to the deceased

Preoccupation with feelings of worthlessness

Psychomotor retardation

Prolonged and marked functional impairment

Hallucinatory experiences (other than image or voice of deceased)

One month after bereavement approximately one third of bereaved spouses will meet the criteria for a depressive episode. This figure falls to one quarter at 2–7 months and 15 % at 13 months.

In *delayed grief*, symptoms are not manifest for more than two weeks after the bereavement. Delayed grief is said to occur more commonly in response to a sudden or unexpected death. *Inhibited grief* occurs when there is an absence of normal features of the grief reaction and may be associated with feelings of anger or guilt towards the deceased. *Prolonged grief* is defined as grief lasting for more than six months. Whilst the concept is important, six months is an arbitrary cut-off and it is not possible to say exactly when grief ends.

Factors associated with abnormal grief are summarised in Box 3.7.

Box 3.7 Factors predisposing to abnormal grief

Sudden or unexpected death

Suicide or murder

Ambivalent or dependent relationship with deceased

Self-blame

Severe depression

Other concurrent stressful life events

Lower socioeconomic status

Poor social support

Managing grief

Grief is a normal process and each individual will try to come to terms with their loss in a different way. Many will receive support from friends, relatives or spiritual leaders.

Bereavement counselling may be helpful for some, especially in the context of abnormal grief. In the UK, CRUSE (www.crusebereavementcare.org.uk) and Compassionate Friends (www.tcf.org.uk) offer counselling and support for those who have been bereaved.

Benzodiazepines are sometimes used for the short-term management of symptoms of severe autonomic arousal but can inhibit the process of grief. Careful consideration must be given before prescription of these drugs, especially in the elderly population who are at increased risk of side effects. Antidepressants are indicated if the criteria for a depressive disorder are met, as part of a holistic management plan that addresses emotional and social needs.

Suicide

The elderly have a higher risk of completed suicide than any other group worldwide. Suicide in the elderly has not received the amount of attention one would expect considering the high rates of completed versus attempted suicide in this group. This may reflect societal attitudes to aging and the lower economic impact of suicides in older, compared to younger, adults.

Epidemiology

The prevalence of *suicidal ideation* in the elderly is estimated to be as high as 17 %, although results from studies vary depending on criteria used.

Rates of *deliberate self-harm* (attempted suicide, parasuicide) are much lower in the elderly than in the younger population, peaking in the early twenties and then declining steadily to very low rates by the fifties.

Rates of *completed suicide* vary in different countries and cultures and official statistics are probably underestimates. In the UK, evidence must be unequivocal for the coroner to record a verdict of suicide, and recorded rates are lower than for any other western country. Pooled international data shows a steady rise in completed suicide rates with age (Figure 3.1).

The elderly are the highest risk group for completed suicide. The World Health Organisation estimates rates of 50 per 100 000 for men over the age of 75 (15.8 for women). The male to female ratio is 3–4:1, similar to other age groups. Several studies have reported that the increase in suicide rates in the elderly is accounted for almost entirely by men, and that risk is particularly high in elderly white men.

Risk factors

The ratio of completed suicide to deliberate self-harm is much higher in elderly people than in younger adults. This is believed to reflect a higher degree of intent in suicidal

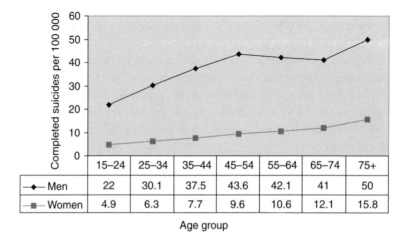

Age group	15–24	25–34	35–44	45–54	55–64	65–74	75+
Men	22	30.1	37.5	43.6	42.1	41	50
Women	4.9	6.3	7.7	9.6	10.6	12.1	15.8

Figure 3.1   Global rates of suicide by age group, 2000. World Health Organisation data

behaviour in the elderly. Older people are more likely to use lethal means, including firearms and hanging.

Psychiatric illness

Depression is more common in elderly suicides than in those of younger adults and is present in up to 83 %. Overall, 71–95 % of elderly people who complete suicide have a psychiatric illness. Increased rates of suicide in personality disorder in the elderly have not been demonstrated, although studies are limited.

Physical illness

Several studies have demonstrated that serious physical illness (e.g. sensory impairment, neurological disorders and malignant disease) is an independent risk factor for suicide in the elderly. However, the effects of physical illness may be mediated by psychiatric illness in some cases.

Social factors

Stressful life events including *bereavement* increase the risk of suicide, as do *social isolation* and *poor social support*. Widowed, single and divorced elderly people have higher rates of suicide than those who are married and whose spouse is alive. Marriage, religion, spiritual well-being and life-satisfaction appear to be protective.

Box 3.8   Risk factors for suicide in the elderly

Depression

Other psychiatric illness

Bereavement

Physical illness

Alcohol

Poor social support

Social isolation

Access to means

Prevention of suicide in the elderly

Of elderly people who complete suicide 40–70 % see their GP in the month before and 20–50 % in the week before the event. The ability of healthcare professionals to recognise at-risk individuals is therefore crucial. Older people are less likely than younger adults to talk about suicidal feelings and it is important to use opportunities to specifically ask those who might be at risk.

General and effective measures to reduce suicide rates include limiting access to means at a population level, for example reducing the number of paracetamol tablets that can be bought over the counter.

Strategies to minimise suicide risk in the elderly include:

• Recognition and treatment of depression and other psychiatric illness

• Optimal treatment of physical illness

• Interventions to improve social contact and support.

Further reading

Depression and bipolar affective disorder

Alexopoulos GS (2005) Depression in the elderly *Lancet* 365: 1961–1970.

Camus V, Kraehenbühl H, Preisig M, Büla CJ and Waeber G (2004) Geriatric depression and vascular diseases: what are the links? *J Affect Disorders* 81(1): 1 –16.

Gebretsadik M, Jayaprabhu S and Grossberg GT (2006) Mood disorders in the elderly *Med Clin N Am* 90: 789–805.

Lyketsos CG and Olin J (2002) Depression in Alzheimer's disease: overview and treatment *Biol Psychiat* 52: 243–252.

Mottram P, Wilson K and Strobl J (2006) Antidepressants for depressed elderly *Cochrane Database Syst Rev* 1: CD003491.

Ranga K and Krishnan R (2002) Biological risk factors in late life depression *Biol Psychiat* 52:185–192.

Bereavement

Clark A (2004) Working with grieving adults *Adv Psychiat Treat* 10: 164–170.

Parkes CM (1965) Bereavement and mental illness. A classification of bereavement reactions *Brit J Med Psychol* 38: 13–26.

Prigerson H, Ellen F, Stanislav V *et al.* (1995) Complicated grief and bereavement-related depression as distinct disorders: preliminary empirical validation in elderly bereaved spouses *Am J Psychiat* 152(1): 22–30.

Rosenzweig A, Prigerson H, Miller M and Reynolds C (1997) Bereavement and late-life depression: grief and its complications in the elderly *Ann Rev Med* 48: 421–428.

Suicide

Heisel MJ (2006) Suicide and its prevention among older adults *Can J Psychiat* 51:143–154.

O'Connell H, Chin AV, Cunningham C and Lawlor BA (2004) Recent developments: suicide in older people *BMJ* 329: 895–899.

4

Bipolar Affective Disorder

Elderly people with bipolar affective disorder (BPAD) fall into two groups. The largest group is made up of those who have a history of bipolar affective disorder that dates back to earlier adulthood. A smaller but significant group is formed by those who first present in old age. In this group, a substantial number will have underlying organic and neurological conditions, and the term *secondary mania* is sometimes used in these cases. Whilst the presentation, course and management of bipolar affective disorder are broadly similar in younger and older adults, there are important features and challenges that are specific to the elderly.

Epidemiology

Only 10 % of all cases of bipolar affective disorder present after the age of 50. Many patients presenting with their first manic episode in old age will have had a depressive episode in middle or late life. The one-year prevalence rate in those aged 18–44 is 1.4 %, decreasing to 0.4 % in the 45–64 years group and 0.1 % in the over 65s. Hospital admission is more common in bipolar affective disorder in old age, accounting for 5–12 % of inpatient admissions despite the low community prevalence. The male:female ratio in the elderly is 2:1.

The Old Age Psychiatry Handbook   Joanne Rodda, Niall Boyce, and Zuzana Walker
© 2008 John Wiley & Sons, Ltd

Table 4.1 Drugs that may induce mania

Antidepressants	Most antidepressants both during and on withdrawing treatment
Antiparkinsonian drugs	Levodopa, bromocriptine, amantidine
Steroids	Most steroid drugs have the potential to induce mania
Cardiovascular drugs	Captopril, methyldopa, clonidine, propanolol, digoxin, diltiazem
Antibiotics	Clarithromycin, drugs used in TB
Analgesics	Opiates, tramadol, buprenorphine, indomethacin
Antiemetics	Cyclizine, metoclopramide
H_2 receptor antagonists	Cimetidine, ranitidine
Other drugs	Baclofen, chloriquine, interferon, cyclosporin

Aetiology

Aetiological factors for bipolar affective disorder in the general adult population include genetic predisposition, drug misuse, personality factors (cyclothymic personality), poor social support and certain adverse childhood experiences. The neurotransmitters serotonin, noradrenaline and dopamine have all been implicated, as have theories involving abnormal programmed cell death and electrophysiological kindling.

The aetiology of late-onset bipolar disorder has been less extensively investigated although there are likely to be similarities. Elderly people who present with their first episode of mania have a high chance of underlying neurological disorder (e.g. stroke, space-occupying lesions, infections, head trauma). As patients grow older, the probability of an organic cause increases and the likelihood of a positive family history for affective disorder decreases.

There is evidence that subtle cerebrovascular changes may contribute to mania in later life in much the same way as in depressive episodes (page 64). MRI scans in elderly patients with mania show a high prevalence of deep white matter and subcortical ischaemic changes, which may be of etiological importance.

Mania can be induced by a number of different drugs (Table 4.1). This is of particular relevance in the elderly population given the increased number of medications prescribed and the increased likelihood of adverse effects.

Clinical features and diagnosis

ICD-10 and DSM-IV have slightly different approaches to the diagnosis of bipolar affective disorder, summarised in Boxes 4.1 and 4.2.

Box 4.1 CD-10 diagnosis of bipolar affective disorder

Two or more episodes of affective disturbance, either:

- episodes of both depression and mania or hypomania

- repeated episodes of mania or hypomania

Box 4.2 DSM-IV diagnosis of bipolar affective disorder

Bipolar 1 disorder

Either:

- at least one episode each of mania and depression or

- multiple manic episodes or

- one manic episode (bipolar 1 disorder, single manic episode)

Bipolar 2 disorder

- episodes of both hypomania and depression

Mania and hypomania

In mania, mood is elevated and there is usually inflated self-esteem, grandiosity and exaggerated optimism. Energy levels are increased, speech is often fast and pressured and sleep is reduced. There is often a lack of normal inhibitions, and individuals may spend large amounts of money, engage in reckless behaviour or make amorous or sexual advances that are out of character. Colours may appear more vividly and there may be a preoccupation with fine detail and textures. There is often marked distractibility and some individuals may present with disorientation, confusion, irritability or aggression.

Some studies have suggested a lesser severity of symptoms in the elderly but evidence is limited. Overall, the clinical picture of mania in the elderly appears very similar to that in younger adults. The clinical impression is that elderly patients present more frequently with mixed affective symptoms.

Psychotic features

Psychotic features are common in mania. Delusions are usually consistent with the patient's mood and often grandiose in nature. Similarly, hallucinations often take the form of voices talking about the patient's special powers. There appears to be no difference in the frequency of psychotic features associated with mania in younger and older adults.

Hypomania

The difference between hypomania and mania is mainly one of degree. Hypomanic patients have many of the same symptoms as manic patients (except psychotic features) but daily life is not completely disrupted.

Diagnostic criteria

The DSM-IV criteria for mania are very similar to ICD-10 (Box 4.3). For hypomania ICD-10 requires symptoms to be present for four consecutive days with less impairment of personal function in daily living and no psychotic features.

Box 4.3 ICD-10 diagnostic criteria for mania

Symptoms for at least one week

Elevated, expansive or irritable mood

At least 3 of:

- ⇑ activity or physical restlessness

- grandiosity or ⇑ self-esteem

- increased talkativeness

- distractibility

- flight of ideas or racing thoughts

- reckless behaviour

- social disinhibition

- increased sexual energy

- decreased need for sleep

Symptoms cause severe interference with personal functioning in daily living

---

Mixed affective states and rapid cycling

In a mixed affective state, symptoms of both mania and depression appear simultaneously, or alternate rapidly. This can present a confusing picture in which a patient with a depressed mood presents as over-talkative and restless. In terms of diagnosis of bipolar affective disorder, mixed affective episodes carry the same weight as manic episodes in ICD-10 and DSM-IV. The clinical impression is that elderly patients present more frequently with mixed affective symptoms.

Patients with rapid cycling bipolar affective disorder have four or more affective episodes in 12 months and may be less responsive to drug treatment.

Cognitive impairment

Cognitive impairment in depression is associated with an increased risk of dementia (page 61). In elderly manic patients there are often impairments in memory and other cognitive domains (attention, executive functioning, psychomotor speed). These deficits may persist after resolution of the affective symptoms but their long-term significance is unclear.

Differential diagnosis

The differential diagnosis of bipolar affective disorder includes other psychiatric as well as organic diagnoses. Elderly people with mania and no previous manic episodes often have an underlying neurological or other physical disorder. It is essential that these patients undergo full investigation (see Chapter 1), including neuroimaging.

Table 4.2   Differential diagnosis of bipolar affective disorder

Psychiatric	Schizoaffective disorder
	Schizophrenia
	Personality disorder
Neurological	Delirium
	Tumour
	Head injury
	CNS infection, e.g. encephalitis
	Cerebrovascular disease
	Multiple sclerosis
Endocrine	Thyroid dysfunction
	Hyperparathyroidism
	Cushing's/Addison's disease
	Hypoglycaemia
Systemic disorder	Hepatic/renal failure
	Rheumatological disorder e.g. SLE (see Chapter 14)
	Malignancy
Nutritional deficits	Folate
	Vitamin B12
	Thiamine
Drugs	Psychoactive substance misuse

Management

There are few randomised controlled trials of specific drugs in the management of bipolar affective disorder in the elderly. Practice is generally guided by small, non-randomised trials, naturalistic studies, studies of mixed age groups, extrapolations from studies of younger patients and clinical experience.

Lithium

Lithium (page 179) is widely used as a first line treatment in the elderly in acute mania and in prophylaxis of manic and depressive episodes. It has a narrow therapeutic window and requires careful monitoring. Given the reduced renal clearance in the elderly, doses are lower than for younger adults. The target serum lithium level is also lower in the elderly, who often develop toxicity when levels are in the "therapeutic" range for younger adults.

Anticonvulsants

Valproate

Valproate (page 184) is widely used in the treatment of acute mania and also in prophylaxis of affective episodes. There is no evidence that it is superior to lithium or antipsychotics in elderly bipolar patients but it is generally well tolerated in older people. Based on its side-effect profile, valproate may be preferable in some older patients.

Valproate may have a role in augmentation of lithium therapy, enabling lower doses of lithium to be used with comparable clinical effect. It may also be more effective than lithium in treating mania that occurs in the context of rapid cycling or an underlying neurological or physical disorder.

Carbamazepine

Carbamazepine (page 185) is effective in the treatment of acute mania and prophylaxis of mania and depression. However, it may be less effective than lithium in long-term treatment and less effective than valproate in acute mania (based on studies of mixed age populations).

Carbamazepine has complex pharmacokinetic interactions with other drugs and induces its own metabolism. In general its side-effect profile is less favourable than valproate, with potential for agranulocytosis and cardiotoxic and neurotoxic effects.

Lamotrigine, gabapentin and topiramate

Lamotrigine may be more effective than other drugs in preventing depressive relapses but it is not currently licensed for use in bipolar affective disorder in the UK and there are few data available concerning its use in the elderly. Gabapentin and topiramate have also been used but evidence regarding their efficacy is limited and they are not licensed for this purpose in the UK.

Antipsychotics

Antipsychotic drugs are widely used in the treatment of mania in young adults. The elderly are more susceptible to side effects than younger people. Concerns regarding their use include:

- Extrapyramidal side effects

- Weight gain and diabetes

- Sedation

- Hypotension

- Precipitation of depressive episode.

Risperidone, olanzapine, quetiapine and aripiprazole all appear to be effective in treating mania but there are few studies of their use in elderly manic patients. Quetiapine may be effective whilst causing few extrapyramidal side effects. Aripiprazole has not been studied in mania in the elderly.

Benzodiazepines

Low doses of short acting benzodiazepines (e.g. lorazepam, page 193) may be necessary to manage agitation or behavioural disturbances associated with affective episodes. In the elderly the use of benzodiazepines is kept to a minimum and potential benefits are balanced against the risk of sedation, confusion and falls.

Antidepressants

Depressive episodes in bipolar affective disorder are treated with antidepressants but caution is necessary as they may precipitate mania. A mood stabiliser is used simultaneously and the antidepressant is usually withdrawn on resolution of depressive symptoms.

How long to treat for? Prophylaxis in bipolar affective disorder

The issue of prophylactic pharmacological treatment in elderly bipolar patients has not been studied in detail. NICE guidelines for young adults recommend treatment for two years after an episode of bipolar affective disorder and five years if patients are at high risk of relapse (history of frequent relapses, social stress, severe psychotic features). Many believe that older people with bipolar affective disorder benefit from long-term prophylactic pharmacotherapy.

Psychological treatment

Psychological therapies may be of benefit in bipolar affective disorder after resolution of the acute episode. Cognitive behavioural therapy and family interventions (page 213) may be useful adjuncts to prophylactic medication. Therapy may focus on strategies to maintain remission (e.g. adherence, regular routines), to identify the "early warning" signs of a manic or depressive episode (relapse signature), and to recognise and cope with affective symptoms.

ECT

ECT (page 206) is sometimes used in the treatment of severe or prolonged manic or depressive episodes where other treatments have not been effective or where the condition is life-threatening.

Managing acute mania and hypomania

NICE guidelines for management of bipolar affective disorder (Figure 4.1) in adults and are helpful when considering management of elderly patients. An approach to managing bipolar affective disorder in older people is given in Table 4.3. The principles of management of acute behavioural disturbance in mania are similar to those in dementia (see Table 2.8, page 32).

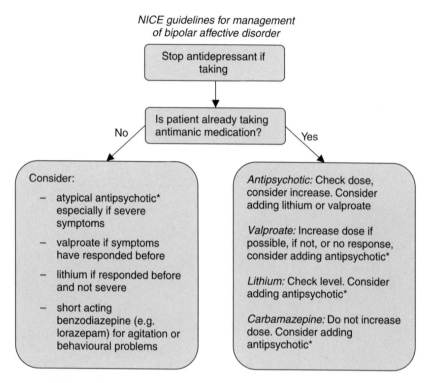

Figure 4.1 NICE guidelines for management of acute mania or hypomania in adults
*NICE recommend olanzapine, risperidone or quetiapine

Course and prognosis

Overall mortality is increased in elderly people with BPAD. Admissions may occur more frequently and it seems that manic episodes are followed more rapidly by depressive episodes. There is little data available regarding the natural history of late-onset bipolar affective disorder but outcome will be dependent at least in part on adherence to medication and appropriate treatment of co-morbid medical conditions.

Table 4.3 An approach to pharmacological management of bipolar affective disorder in the elderly

Indication	First line pharmacological treatments
Manic, hypomanic or mixed episode	Lithium/valproate/atypical antipsychotic
Depressive episode	Antidepressant and mood stabiliser. Stop antidepressant when symptoms resolve
Rapid cycling	Valproate with or without lithium
Prophylaxis	Lithium/valproate

5

Anxiety Disorders and Obsessive Compulsive Disorder

Anxiety in the elderly

Anxiety disorders are common in the elderly but often go unrecognised and untreated. Although initial reports suggested a decline in prevalence with age, more recent studies have found that this might not be the case. Anxiety in the elderly is often a presenting feature of depression and sometimes of dementia. It is also a common symptom in many other psychiatric disorders. Distinguishing symptoms of anxiety (Table 5.1) from those of physical illness is a particularly important consideration in older people.

The Old Age Psychiatry Handbook Joanne Rodda, Niall Boyce, and Zuzana Walker
© 2008 John Wiley & Sons, Ltd

Table 5.1   Clinical features of anxiety

Mental state	Autonomic arousal	Other
Worry	Increased heart rate	Sleep disturbance
Apprehension	Palpitations	Irritability
Poor concentration	Hyperventilation	Exaggerated startle response
Fear of:	Tremor	Obsessions
– losing control	Sweating	
– dying	Nausea	
– passing out	Dry mouth	
– "going crazy"	Chest/epigastric discomfort	
Depersonalisation	Dizziness	
Derealisation	Frequent micturition	

Epidemiology

Differences in diagnostic criteria and case definition mean that estimates of prevalence of anxiety disorders in the elderly vary between approximately 5–10 %. Rates are highest among the housebound, nursing home residents, older medical patients and those with chronic illness.

Anxiety and physical health

The relationship between anxiety and physical illness is complex:

- Anxiety disorders and physical illness are both common in the elderly and may occur simultaneously.

- Physical ill-health is a source of anxiety for many people.

- Many physical illnesses directly cause anxiety symptoms (Table 5.2 gives common examples).

- Symptoms of anxiety can be mistaken for those of physical illness.

Drugs

Many drugs can cause symptoms of anxiety, including over-the-counter medications, alcohol and caffeine (Box 5.1). Withdrawal from drugs is also an important consideration.

Table 5.2 Physical conditions that commonly cause anxiety symptoms

Cardiovascular	Heart failure Angina Myocardial infarction Arrhythmias
Respiratory	Chronic obstructive airways disease/asthma Pneumonia Pulmonary embolism
Neurological	Parkinson's disease Stroke Many other neurological disorders
Endocrine	Hyperthyroidism Cushing's Phaeochromocytoma Hypoglycaemia

---

Box 5.1 Drugs that commonly cause anxiety symptoms

Alcohol

Caffeine

Sympathomimetics in over-the-counter medications

Steroids

Thyroxine

Anticholinergics

Antidepressants

Co-morbid anxiety and depression

Symptoms of anxiety are often associated with depression. It can be difficult to differentiate between the two disorders and there is a great deal of overlap in symptomatology. Older people may find it hard to explain the feeling of low mood and may find it easier to talk about their "nerves". It may be that elderly people presenting with anxiety are more likely than younger patients with a similar presentation to have an underlying depressive illness.

When anxiety is associated with depression in older adults there is:

• A greater severity of depressive symptoms

- An increased likelihood of suicidal ideation

- Lower social functioning

- A negative impact on remission of depressive episode.

Many older patients have co-morbid depressive and anxious symptoms that do not meet the criteria for an anxiety disorder or a depressive episode. These patients experience significant distress and functional impairment, which may be more severe than for those with anxiety disorder alone. SSRIs or psychological therapy may be beneficial in these cases although there is no specific evidence.

Generalised anxiety disorder

Generalised anxiety disorder (GAD) is the most common anxiety disorder in older adults. Community prevalence estimates amongst the elderly range from 1.9–7.3 %. Around half of patients have had symptoms for most of their lives whilst in the other half the onset of GAD is in old age. At all ages GAD is more common in women than men.

Clinical features and diagnosis

Symptoms of anxiety (Table 5.1) are present almost all of the time although there may be variations in intensity. Worry is generalised and not centred on one specific subject, and there is usually a feeling of not being in control. Diagnostic criteria are summarised in Boxes 5.2 and 5.3. There appears to be no difference in symptomatology between younger and older adults.

Box 5.2   ICD-10 criteria for diagnosis of generalised anxiety disorder

At least six months with prominent tension, worry and feelings of apprehension about everyday events and problems

At least four symptoms of anxiety from a specified list. Symptoms usually involve elements of:

- tension, worry and feelings of apprehension about everyday issues

- autonomic overactivity

- motor tension

Criteria for panic, phobic anxiety or obsessive compulsive disorders not met

---

Box 5.3 DSM-IV criteria for diagnosis of generalised anxiety disorder

Excessive anxiety and worry for more than half of the days for at least six months

Difficult to control the worry

At least three of the following also present:

   −restlessness, feeling edgy or keyed up

   −increased fatiguability

   −difficulty concentrating

   −irritability

   −muscle tension

   −insomnia

Symptoms not accounted for by another physical or psychiatric disorder and cause distress or impair function

Does not occur only during a mood disorder, psychotic disorder or post-traumatic stress disorder

---

Management

Pharmacological

The high rate of depressive co-morbidity in GAD in the elderly supports the use of medications with both anxiolytic and antidepressant effects.

Antidepressants are probably the treatment of choice. Studies in older adults are limited but citalopram and venlafaxine have been shown to be effective and well tolerated.

Benzodiazepines (page 193) are effective in treating the symptoms of anxiety but at the cost of confusion, sedation, falls, tolerance and dependence. Use of benzodiazepines is limited to low doses for short periods and is generally avoided.

Buspirone has been shown to be effective in the treatment of GAD and does not cause sedation or dependence. It may be less effective than antidepressants in the treatment of

GAD in the elderly. Buspirone may be less effective in individuals who have previously taken a benzodiazepine, which will be the case for many elderly patients with GAD.

Pregabalin is an anticonvulsant drug that has recently been licensed for use in GAD. One large RCT supports its efficacy and tolerability in elderly patients.

Beta-blockers are sometimes prescribed to treat the physiological symptoms of anxiety but in elderly patients the benefit is likely to be outweighed by the risk of side effects.

Non-pharmacological

CBT is effective in elderly patients with GAD but less so than in younger adults. Nondirective supportive therapy may be as effective as CBT in the elderly.

Course and prognosis

GAD in younger adults tends to run a chronic course. However, GAD with onset in later life appears to have higher rates of remission, which may be linked to the association with depressive episodes. The duration of pharmacological therapy may therefore be guided by the need for maintenance treatment of depression.

Panic disorder

Panic disorder affects 0.1–1 % of older adults although onset in old age is uncommon. The peak age of onset is usually in early adulthood; symptoms sometimes run a chronic course into old age. The symptoms of panic disorder may be less severe in the elderly than in younger adults.

Clinical features and diagnosis

A *panic attack* is an episode of extreme anxiety (Table 5.1) that develops rapidly and usually lasts several minutes. *Panic disorder* is the repeated occurrence of panic attacks, in the absence of a specific cause (e.g. physical illness, another psychiatric diagnosis, substance misuse).

DSM-IV criteria are very similar to ICD-10 (Box 5.4), although in DSM-IV panic disorder is classified as occurring with or without agoraphobia (below).

> **Box 5.4 ICD-10 criteria for panic disorder**
>
> Recurrent attacks of severe anxiety not consistently restricted to a particular situation
>
> Several attacks within a period of about one month
>
> — in situations with no obvious danger
>
> — not confined to known or predictable situations
>
> — relatively free from anxiety in between attacks
>
> Panic attacks must not be the result of another psychiatric or physical disorder

Co-morbidity

Panic attacks occur as a part of many psychiatric disorders. Panic attacks secondary to *depression* are particularly common. Panic symptoms may be severe enough to eclipse depressive features and depression may consequently go unrecognised. Some medical conditions are particularly associated with panic, including chronic obstructive airways disease.

Management

Again, antidepressants are the mainstay of pharmacological treatment, with *SSRIs* being the first choice. Recognition and management of co-morbid conditions is crucial. *Cognitive behavioural therapy* in panic disorder has not been extensively investigated in the elderly but the evidence available supports its efficacy.

Course

Panic disorder is usually a chronic syndrome with frequent relapses and remissions. The majority of elderly patients will have suffered from panic disorder for many years; there are few data available regarding the continued course of the disorder.

Phobic disorders

Phobic disorders are relatively common in the elderly although onset is usually in early life. Estimates of prevalence in older adults range from 0.7–13.4 %. This variability is largely accounted for by the wide range of prevalence estimates for agoraphobia. Prevalence is higher in women than in men except in social phobia.

Clinical features

Unreasonably severe symptoms of anxiety occur in response to (or in anticipation of) specific objects or situations. The individual avoids the objects or situations that provoke the anxiety. Phobic disorders in the elderly have been shown to be associated with increased psychiatric and medical morbidity compared to controls.

Agoraphobia

Patients with agoraphobia experience anxiety in situations where escape might be difficult or embarrassing, resulting in avoidance (e.g. crowds, public transport). Older people may develop symptoms of agoraphobia with increasing physical frailty. Estimates of prevalence in the elderly range from 1.4 to 7.9 %.

In DSM-IV (Box 5.6), agoraphobia is not coded as a disorder in its own right, but rather as a part of other disorders (e.g. panic disorder with agoraphobia). In ICD-10 (Box 5.5), agoraphobia is coded as occurring with or without panic disorder.

Box 5.5   ICD-10 criteria for agoraphobia

Marked and consistently manifest fear in, or avoidance of, two or more of:

– crowds

– public places

– travelling away from home

– travelling alone

Significant emotional distress is caused by the avoidance or by the anxiety symptoms

Symptoms are restricted to, or predominate in, the feared situations or contemplation of the feared situations

---

Box 5.6 DSM-IV criteria for agoraphobia

The individual fears situations in which one or both of the following may occur:

- escape could be difficult or embarrassing

- help might not be available in the event of a panic attack

The individual responds in one of the following ways:

- avoids these situations/places

- does not avoid but suffers distress (e.g. panic attack)

- requires a companion

Symptoms are not better explained by another mental disorder

Box 5.7 ICD-10 criteria for social phobia

Either of the following must be present in social situations:

- fear of being focus of attention or of behaving in an embarrassing/humiliating way

- avoidance of the above or situations that may lead to this

General symptoms of anxiety occur in the feared situation plus at least one of:

- blushing or shaking

- fear of vomiting

- urgency or fear of micturition or defaecation

Significant emotional distress is caused by the avoidance or by the anxiety symptoms

Symptoms are restricted to, or predominate in, the feared situations or contemplation of the feared situations

---

Box 5.8   DSM-IV criteria for social phobia

Fear of one or more social situations

Fear of showing anxiety or behaving in an embarrassing or humiliating way

The phobic situation almost always causes anxiety

Situations are either avoided or endured with distress

Marked distress about having the phobia or interference with functioning

Symptoms are not better explained by another mental or physical disorder

---

Social phobia

Social phobia usually has onset in young adulthood and runs a chronic course. Prevalence in the elderly is around 1 % and is equal in men and women. There is anxiety in social situations, particularly in small groups, leading to avoidance of these situations. Individuals may fear acting in a way that is humiliating or embarrassing, or that others will notice their anxiety.

Specific phobias

Specific phobias are restricted to particular objects or situations. Onset is usually in childhood but phobias can persist for many years if not adequately treated. Prevalence estimates in older adults range from 3.1 to 12 %. Older people are more likely to report phobias of lightning, heights and flying compared to younger adults whose phobias more often include spiders and injections.

The diagnostic criteria for specific phobia are very similar to those for social phobia, except that anxiety is restricted to the presence of a different specific phobic object or situation.

Management

It is quite unusual for people to seek treatment for phobic disorders in old age. The mainstay of treatment is psychological. Behavioural methods (page 216) involve exposure to the feared stimulus, for example graded exposure with relaxation. CBT, anxiety management and development of coping skills can also be beneficial.

Strategies for pharmacological management are mainly based on studies of younger adults and tolerability of medications in older adults. In agoraphobia or social phobia SSRIs are the first choice if medication is to be used, particularly if there are associated depressive features. Medication is rarely indicated in specific phobias.

Post-traumatic stress disorder

Post-traumatic stress disorder (PTSD) is a response to an event of an extremely traumatic or catastrophic nature. Symptoms usually arise after one month, but within six months of the event. The central feature is intrusive recollection of the traumatic event in the form of vivid memories, flashbacks or recurring dreams. There is psychological or physiological hyperarousal and the individual avoids situations that resemble the traumatic event (Boxes 5.9 and 5.10). Co-morbid depression, anxiety and alcohol or other substance misuse are common.

Box 5.9   ICD-10 diagnostic criteria for post-traumatic stress disorder

Exposure to a stressful situation of exceptionally threatening or catastrophic nature, which would be likely to cause pervasive stress in almost anyone

Symptoms usually arise within six months of the event

Repetitive, intrusive recollection or re-enactment of the event in flashbacks, vivid memories or recurring dreams

Avoidance of situations associated with the stressor

One or both of the following must be present:

1. Inability to recall important aspects of the period of exposure to the stressor

2. Psychological sensitivity and arousal shown by two of:

   – irritability/angry outbursts

   – poor concentration

   – hypervigilance

   – exaggerated startle response

Box 5.10   DSM-IV criteria for post-traumatic stress disorder (brief summary)

Exposure to an unusually traumatic event and:

- – the event involved actual or threatened death or serious injury to the patient or others, and

- – the patient felt intense fear, horror or hopelessness

Repeated reliving of the event through thoughts, images, dreams, flashbacks, hallucinations, illusions; or distress in reaction to cues that trigger recollection of the trauma

Numbing of general responsiveness and avoidance of stimuli related to the trauma

Symptoms of hyperarousal that were not present before the traumatic event

Symptoms present for more than one month and cause distress or impair functioning

---

The rates of PTSD following a disaster are probably similar for younger and older adults. However, older people who are physically frail or who have cognitive impairment may feel more threatened in some situations than younger adults.

There is some evidence that PTSD symptoms may re-emerge or become apparent for the first time after an extended delay in elderly people. Studies of Second World War and Korean War veterans have suggested that PTSD symptoms peak soon after the exposure, after which they gradually decline but then increase again in old age.

Management

There is little specific evidence upon which to base decisions regarding the management of PTSD in older adults. Cognitive behavioural therapy is widely used in younger adults. There is less evidence for eye movement desensitisation and reprocessing.

SSRIs, tricyclic antidepressants and mirtazapine have been shown to have efficacy in PTSD. However, effect sizes are smaller than for psychological therapy and so drug treatment is not recommended as first line by NICE (Box 5.11).

> **Box 5.11   NICE guidelines for management of PTSD**
>
> Consider screening for all people involved in a major disaster at one month
>
> Consider watchful waiting if symptoms are mild and present for less than four weeks
>
> All those with PTSD symptoms in the month after the trauma should be offered CBT
>
> All PTSD sufferers should be offered trauma-focused psychological treatment
>
> Drug treatment should not be first line. Consider paroxetine, TCAs or mirtazapine if psychological therapy is not acceptable to the patient

Other reactions to stress

Acute stress reaction

An acute stress reaction is a transient disorder that develops in response to an episode of extreme physical or psychological stress. It may occur in an individual with or without a history of mental disorder.

The individual usually appears "dazed" and this may be followed by depression, anxiety, disorientation, narrowing of attention, aggression, hopelessness and withdrawal. The elderly are more vulnerable to acute stress reactions than younger adults and risk is increased by physical exhaustion and organic disorders. Symptoms are apparent within hours and usually resolve within hours or days; management is supportive.

Adjustment disorders

The core feature in adjustment disorders is a state of subjective distress and emotional disturbance that interferes with functioning and arises during the stage of adaptation to a significant life change or stressful event. Community prevalence is estimated at 5 %. Onset of symptoms is usually within one month of the change or event and duration is usually less than six months.

Adjustment disorders often occur in response to physical illness or disability. Moving into a residential or nursing home and bereavement (page 73) are also especially relevant in the elderly.

Diagnosis

Box 5.12   ICD-10 criteria for adjustment disorder

Onset of symptoms within one month of identifiable psychosocial stressor

Symptoms do not persist for more than six months*

Symptoms or behavioural disturbance of type found in affective or neurotic disorders

Subtypes include:

–brief depressive reaction (mild depressive state, <1 month duration)

–prolonged depressive reaction (mild depressive state, prolonged stressor, duration <2 years)

–mixed anxiety and depressive reaction

*Except in a prolonged depressive reaction

Box 5.13   DSM-IV criteria for adjustment disorder

Onset of emotional or behavioural symptoms within three months of stressor

Either distress exceeding the level that would be expected *or* impairment of function

Symptoms do not meet criteria for an axis I disorder or represent worsening of symptoms of a pre-existing axis I or II disorder

Symptoms are not caused by bereavement

Symptoms do not last longer than six months after the end of the stressor

---

Management

Management will depend on the nature of the stressor, the severity of symptoms and the needs of the individual patient. Approaches include:

- Supportive psychotherapy/counselling
- Social and practical support (e.g. occupational therapy assessment and input, support groups)
- Pharmacological therapy may be indicated for symptoms of anxiety or depression.

Obsessive compulsive disorder

The onset of obsessive compulsive disorder (OCD) is usually before the age of 25; onset after the age of 50 is rare. However, symptoms can run a chronic course into old age, especially in the absence of treatment. Prevalence in elderly populations is unclear.

Clinical features and diagnosis

Obsessions are intrusive thoughts, images or impulses that the individual:

- Experiences as unpleasant

- Tries to resist

- Is aware arise from his own mind.

    A compulsion is a behaviour or act that the individual:

- Is unable to resist performing, usually repeatedly

- Recognises as purposeless

- Experiences a need to perform in order to reduce distress or prevent an unwanted event from happening.

    Patients with OCD experience obsessions and/or compulsions to a degree that interferes with functioning. At some point during the disorder they recognise these symptoms as senseless. Common examples are:

- Checking

- Washing

- Contamination

- Doubting

- Symmetry

- Violent thoughts.

Diagnosis

Box 5.14   ICD-10 criteria for obsessive compulsive disorder

Obsessions and/or compulsions present on most days for at least two weeks

Obsessions and compulsions have all of the following features:

  −acknowledged as originating within the mind of the patient

  −repetitive and unpleasant

  −at least one must be acknowledged as unreasonable

  −patient tries to resist (must be unable to resist at least one)

  −the experience of the obsession or compulsion is not pleasurable

Obsessions or compulsions cause distress or interfere with functioning

Obsessions or compulsions do not arise as a result of another mental disorder

---

DSM-IV criteria are generally similar to ICD-10 although DSM-IV gives more specific definitions of obsessions and compulsions.

Associations and co-morbidity

Patients with OCD often experience depressive episodes, which may be masked by worsening of obsessive-compulsive symptoms. Co-morbidity with other anxiety disorders is common.

Obsessions and compulsions can occur as a feature in depression, anxiety disorders, schizophrenia and dementia. There is also evidence of an increased incidence of obsessive-compulsive symptoms in Parkinson's disease.

Management

There is little specific information available regarding the management of OCD in the elderly. Decisions are based on the needs of the individual patient and recommendations for younger adults.

Psychological therapy

Behavioural therapy involving exposure and response prevention may be beneficial. The role of cognitive therapy is less clear.

Pharmacotherapy

SSRIs and clomipramine are first line drugs. High doses are often needed and the delay in onset of action may be up to 12 weeks. SSRIs are the safest choice in the elderly.

NICE guidelines for the management of OCD are summarised in Box 5.15. Note that combinations of drugs or the use of antipsychotics are less likely to be appropriate in the elderly because of the increased risk of side effects.

Box 5.15 NICE guidelines for management of OCD

Offer CBT, including exposure and response prevention

If CBT is inadequate or patient declines, offer SSRI or SSRI + CBT

If no/inadequate response offer a different SSRI or clomipramine

If still no/inadequate response consider:

   – additional CBT or cognitive therapy

   – adding antipsychotic to SSRI or clomipramine

   – combining clomipramine and citalopram

Further reading

Averill PM (2000) Posttraumatic stress disorder in older adults: a conceptual review *J Anxiety Disord* 14: 133–156.

Flint AJ (2005) Generalised anxiety disorder in elderly patients. Epidemiology, diagnosis and treatment options *Drugs Ageing* 22: 101–114.

Heikh JI and Cassidy EL (2000) Treatment of anxiety disorders in the elderly: issues and strategies *J Anxiety Disord* 14: 173–190.

Krasucki C, Howard R and Mann A (1998) The relationship between anxiety disorders and age *Int J Geriat Psychiat* 13: 79–99.

Lauderdale SA and Sheikh JI (2003) Anxiety disorders in older adults *Clin Geriat Med* 19: 721–741.

Montgomery SA (2006) Pregabalin for the treatment of generalised anxiety disorder *Exp Opin Pharmacother* 7: 2139–2154.

Wetherell JL, Lenze EJ and Stanley MA (2005) Evidence-based treatment of geriatric anxiety disorders *Psychiat Clin N Am* 28: 871–896.

6

Psychotic Illness

Many older adults with psychotic illness, particularly schizophrenia, will have developed the illness in earlier life but some will not have onset of symptoms until old age. There has been considerable debate about whether these groups represent distinct illnesses, and a consensus on nomenclature has only recently been reached.

Schizophrenia

Definitions

A variety of terms have been used to describe the onset of schizophrenia in later life (Box 6.1). The International Late-Onset Schizophrenia Group agreed on the following definitions, published in 2000:

Late-onset schizophrenia: schizophrenia-like illness with onset between age 40 and 60.

Very late onset schizophrenia like psychosis (VLOSLP): schizophrenia-like illness with onset after age 60.

The Old Age Psychiatry Handbook   Joanne Rodda, Niall Boyce, and Zuzana Walker
© 2008 John Wiley & Sons, Ltd

Box 6.1   Terms used for psychotic illness with onset in old age

Paraphrenia

Late paraphrenia

Late-onset schizophrenia

Late life schizophrenia

Late onset schizophrenia-like psychotic illness

Very late onset schizophrenia-like psychotic illness

Epidemiology

Of patients with schizophrenia, 15–20 % have onset after the age of 44, and 3 % over the age of 60. Community prevalence estimates for schizophrenia in those over 65 range from 0.1–0.5 %. Data from first admissions suggest that the annual incidence of schizophrenia-like psychosis increases by 11 % in each five-year age bracket after the age of 60. Late-onset schizophrenia and VLOSLP are significantly more common in women but estimates of ratios vary.

Aetiology and risk factors

The most important risk factors for onset of a schizophrenia-like illness in old age are female gender, sensory impairment and social isolation (Box 6.2).

Box 6.2   Risk factors for very late onset schizophrenia-like psychosis

Female gender

Sensory impairment (hearing > visual)

Social isolation

Abnormal premorbid personality

Poor premorbid social functioning

Abnormal premorbid personality (schizoid or paranoid personality traits) and poor premorbid social functioning have been reported in many patients with later-onset schizophrenia. However, people with late-onset schizophrenia are more likely than those with early onset to have married, had children and worked.

Genetic and neurodevelopmental factors have both been shown to be of importance in the aetiology of early-onset schizophrenia but appear to be of lesser importance in the aetiology of later-onset illness.

Clinical features and diagnosis

Clinical features of schizophrenia

Positive symptoms are delusions and hallucinations. Delusions are generally persecutory, or of thought interference or control. Hallucinations are classically in the form of a third person running commentary or voices discussing the patient.

Negative symptoms include apathy, affective flattening and poverty of speech.

Other symptoms include:

- Thought disorder

- Depression

- Agitation

- Passivity phenomena

- Cognitive impairments (below)

- Soft neurological signs

- Catatonic symptoms (excitement, posturing, waxy flexibility, negativism, mutism, stupor, mannerisms, stereotypy).

Diagnostic criteria

ICD-10 and DSM-IV do not contain separate codes for diagnosis of schizophrenia with onset in late life. The validity of current criteria (Boxes 6.3 and 6.4) for diagnosis of late-onset schizophrenia is unclear, although symptoms are relatively similar (see below).

Box 6.3   Summary of ICD-10 criteria for schizophrenia

At least one of the following present for most of the time for one month:

– thought echo, thought insertion or withdrawal, thought broadcasting

– delusions of control, influence or passivity or delusional perception

– persistent delusions of other kinds that are completely impossible and culturally inappropriate

– auditory hallucinations:

  • running commentary

  • discussing the patient

  • other types of hallucinatory voices coming from some part of the body

Or at least two of the following present for most of the time for one month:

– persistent hallucinations in any modality when accompanied by:

  • delusions without clear affective content

  • persistent over-valued ideas

  • occurrence every day for weeks or months on end

– Neologisms or breaks or interpolations in the chain of thought resulting in incoherence or irrelevant speech

– catatonic behaviour

– negative symptoms

Box 6.4   Summary of DSM-IV criteria for schizophrenia

Two or more of the following present for at least one month (less if treated):

−delusions*

−hallucinations*

−speech that is incoherent or shows derailment or other disorganisation

−severely disorganised or catatonic behaviour

−negative symptoms

In addition, some evidence of the disorder must have been present for at least six
months, evidenced by one or both of:

−negative symptoms

−at least two of the symptoms above in attenuated form

Impairment of function

Symptoms are not due to mood disorder, schizoaffective disorder or physical illness

*Only one symptom is required if delusions are bizarre or if auditory hallucinations are running
commentary or voices discussing the patient

Changes in early-onset schizophrenia with ageing

A number of changes have been reported in the features of early-onset schizophrenia
with ageing:

Positive symptoms tend to persist but it is unusual to develop new delusions or hallucinations in old age.

There is no clear evidence that *negative symptoms* either improve or worsen in old age.

By the time old age is reached, individuals may have developed ways of managing their
illness and life may be less demanding. This may allow development of better coping
strategies and some aspects of social functioning may improve.

Table 6.1 Summary of differences in symptomatology between onset of schizophrenia in old age and in younger adults

	Early onset	Onset in old age
Delusions	Systematised or non-systematised	Systematised, persecutory
Hallucinations	Almost always auditory	Auditory
		Visual
		Olfactory
Thought disorder	Common	Rare
Negative symptoms	Common	Rare

Onset in old age

The symptom profile in later-onset illness is broadly similar to that in early-onset schizophrenia, especially in terms of positive symptoms. There are, however, important differences.

Patients with onset of illness in old age are more likely to experience visual, tactile and olfactory hallucinations, which may be related to specific sensory organ pathology. Persecutory delusions, third person running commentary and accusatory or derogatory auditory hallucinations are also more common.

Persecutory delusions often relate to:

- Transgressions of personal space (e.g. uninvited people in the home)

- Theft

- Jealousy

- Infestation.

Formal thought disorder and negative symptoms are uncommon.

Differential diagnosis

The differential diagnosis of a psychotic illness with onset in old age includes:

- Affective psychosis

- Delusional disorder

- Schizoaffective disorder

- Dementia

- Delirium

- Alcohol (or rarely illicit substance) misuse

- Specific organic cause (e.g. tumour)

Schizophrenia, cognitive impairment and dementia

In early-onset schizophrenia there is usually generalised cognitive impairment with deficits in:

- Memory

- Attention

- Language

- Visuospatial ability

- Executive function.

In general, the cognitive deficits found in later-onset schizophrenia are qualitatively and quantitatively similar to those found in early-onset patients.

The pattern of cognitive deficits found in schizophrenia is different from that found in dementia and individuals with early-onset schizophrenia have similar rates of dementia to the rest of the population. However, there may be a rapid functional decline in this group as they reach their seventies and eighties.

Some have suggested that late-onset schizophrenic illnesses represent a prodromal state of dementia in some patients. This is consistent with very limited evidence of an increased incidence of dementia in this group. However, other evidence does not support this hypothesis:

1. There is no higher genetic loading in later-onset cases for:

   - Alzheimer's disease

   - dementia with Lewy bodies

   - apolipoprotein E ε4.

2. Neuropathological studies have shown that onset of schizophrenia-like illnesses in middle or old age is not associated with obvious amyloid pathology.

Overall, evidence concerning the relationship between schizophrenia and dementia is limited and more specific studies are needed to improve our understanding of this association.

Neuroimaging

Structural neuroimaging findings in later-onset illness are similar to those found in patients with early-onset schizophrenia. There is increased ventricle-to-brain volume ratio, third ventricle enlargement and reduced frontal and temporal lobe or superior temporal gyrus volume. More recent functional imaging studies have failed to consistently demonstrate elevated striatal D2 receptor concentrations.

No excess of focal structural abnormalities or specific cerebrovascular changes has been demonstrated in VLOSLP. One consistent difference is an increase in white matter hyperintensities in later-onset compared to early-onset cases.

Co-morbidity

Elderly patients with schizophrenia appear to have the same rate of physical illness as people of a similar age without a mental illness. However, these illnesses may be more severe, reflecting a poorer standard of healthcare received.

Recognition of co-morbid physical illness is extremely important in older patients with schizophrenia, as they are frequently undiagnosed. People with psychosis may be less likely to access health services, report symptoms and adhere to treatment. This could be due to negative symptoms of psychosis and cognitive impairment (and positive symptoms if symptoms are subject to delusional interpretation). There is also some evidence that increased pain tolerance in people with psychosis may lead to under-reporting of symptoms.

Management

Pharmacological management

Atypical antipsychotics have been shown to have fewer side effects and may have a better clinical effect than typical antipsychotics in older adults with schizophrenia. Most evidence exists for risperidone and olanzapine. The required doses are much lower than for younger adults, sometimes as low as one tenth of the standard dose. Rates of extrapyramidal side effects may be as high as 50 % even at low doses.

Table 6.2 Brief summary of management of schizophrenia in old age

Intervention	Notes
Pharmacological	Atypical antipsychotic drugs. Low doses (as low as 1/10 younger adult dose).
Psychological	Manualised cognitive behavioural therapy/social and functional skills training.
Social	Appropriate support at home, accommodation, benefits etc.
Other	Hearing aids/glasses if required. Admission to hospital will be necessary in some cases. Input from other professionals, e.g. occupational therapist, community psychiatric nurse, social worker. Day centre/hospital.

Antidepressant augmentation with citalopram may improve depression and global functioning. Cholinesterase inhibitors improve cognitive function in patients with co-morbid dementia.

Practical and social interventions

Addressing social isolation through day hospital or day centre referral or other means is often key. Treating reversible causes of eyesight and hearing loss (e.g. ear wax removal) and arranging for hearing aids or glasses can help reduce sensory deprivation, which is often an aetiological factor.

Psychological interventions

Preliminary evidence from several small studies indicates that older people with schizophrenia benefit from cognitive behavioural therapy, which has generally been delivered with social and functional skills training in trials to date.

Outcome

Patients with onset of schizophrenia in old age may have a better response to antipsychotics than younger patients. Remission rates of up to 48–61 % have been reported.

The best predictor of the level of adaptive functioning is the level of social support. The most consistent predictors of abnormal daily functioning in elderly patients with schizophrenia are:

• Cognitive impairment

- Negative symptoms

- Abnormal movements.

Mortality

Deaths from unnatural causes are higher in older people with schizophrenia than in the general older population, but this excess is less marked than for the younger population, in which the mortality rate of people with psychosis is two to four-fold greater than that of the general population.

Schizoaffective disorder

Patients with schizoaffective disorder have features of schizophrenia as well as prominent mood symptoms (Box 6.5). Both manic and depressive subtypes of schizoaffective disorder exist, the depressive subtype tends to run a more chronic course.

Box 6.5   Diagnosis of schizoaffective disorder

ICD-10: Schizophrenic and affective symptoms present simultaneously and equally prominent

DSM-IV criteria are more strict:

−symptoms meeting criteria for an affective episode occur concurrently with schizophrenic symptoms for two weeks

−delusions or hallucinations occur for two weeks without prominent mood symptoms

−symptoms meeting criteria for affective episode present for a significant proportion of active and residual phases of the illness

---

Adults with schizoaffective disorder in early life may "graduate" into old age psychiatry. There is very little literature devoted to the possibility of the onset of a similar disorder in old age. The international consensus agreement used the term "very late onset schizophrenia-like psychosis" to describe schizophrenia-like illnesses with onset in old age, and did not distinguish between patients with and without prominent mood symptoms.

Management of schizoaffective disorder is similar to schizophrenia, but the principles of treatment of bipolar affective disorder apply to the management of mood symptoms.

Delusional disorder

Patients with delusional disorder have circumscribed non-bizarre delusions that are persistent and sometimes lifelong. Persecutory delusions are most common; others listed in DSM-IV are somatic, grandiose, erotomanic and jealous. Assessment of risk is particularly important in delusions of infidelity, where there is a significant risk of violence.

Epidemiology

The mean age of onset is 40–49 years and overall prevalence is estimated at 0.025–0.3 % and over 65 at 0.04 %. Many cases with onset in middle age will persist into old age; new-onset cases may be less common.

Incidence is slightly more common in women than men, although delusions of infidelity are more common in men.

Aetiology and risk factors

Risk factors in the elderly have not been specifically investigated but based on studies of younger adults the following are probably important:

- Social isolation

- Low socioeconomic status

- Sensory impairment (especially deafness)

- Family history of delusional disorder or paranoid personality disorder

- Head injury

- Premorbid paranoid personality disorder.

Clinical features

Onset may be sudden or gradual. Individuals function without marked behavioural or emotional disturbance outside of the context of their delusions and there is no cognitive impairment. There may be surprisingly little emotional response to the content of the delusion. Significant depressive symptoms exist in approximately one third of patients.

Diagnostic criteria

Box 6.6   ICD-10 criteria for delusional disorder

Delusion or set of delusions that is not typically schizophrenic*

Present for at least three months

General criteria for schizophrenia are not fulfilled

No persistent hallucinations in any modality

Depressive symptoms may be present intermittently but delusions must also be
   present at other times

Not due to other medical or psychiatric disorder or drug use

*See Box 6.3

DSM-IV criteria are similar to ICD-10 but require symptoms to have been present
for only one month and for there to be little effect on behaviour and functioning that is
not directly related to the delusion(s). It also specifies subtypes (see above).

Management

Pimozide has historically been used in the treatment of delusional disorder but there is
no RCT evidence to support its use and it is also cardiotoxic. An atypical antipsychotic
is the drug of choice. Antidepressants are often used although their role is unclear. Given
the high rate of depressive symptomatology, it is possible that many patients may benefit.

Psychological therapy may be effective, particularly CBT focused on the delusional
belief.

Outcome

Acute onset of symptoms is associated with better prognosis. Overall there is complete
remission in 33–50 %, noted improvement in 10 % and persisting delusions in 33–50 %.
Prognosis is less favourable when symptoms have been present for more than six months.
Symptoms often recur when medication is stopped; long-term treatment is necessary in
many cases.

Further reading

Cohen CI, Cohen GD, Blank K *et al.* (2000) Schizophrenia and older adults. An overview: directions for research and policy *Am J Gerait Psychiat* 8: 19–28.

Folsom DP, Lebowitz BD, Lindamer LA *et al.* (2006) Schizophrenia in late life: emerging issues *Dial Clin Neurosci* 8: 45–52.

Hassett A, Ames D and Chiu E (2005) *Psychosis in the Elderly* London, Taylor and Francis.

Howard R, Rabins PV, Seeman MV and Jeste DV (2000) Late onset schizophrenia and very late onset schizophrenia-like psychosis: an international consensus *Am J Psychiat* 157: 172–178.

Marriott RG, Neil W and Waddingham S (2006) Antipsychotic medication for elderly people with schizophrenia *Cochrane Database Syst Rev* 1: CD005580.

Van Citters AD, Pratt SI, Bartels SJ and Jeste DV (2005) Evidence-based review of pharmacologic and nonpharmacologic treatments for older adults with schizophrenia *Psychiat Clin N Am* 28: 913–939.

7

Personality Disorders

There is a great disparity between the impact of personality disorders in clinical practice in old age psychiatry and the literature devoted to the subject. Personality disorders are in fact relatively common in old age and have important implications in terms of co-morbidity, outcome of treatment, service provision and therapeutic alliance.

Personality

Personality describes the enduring characteristics of an individual, manifest in their attitudes and behaviour in different situations. In general, personality is developed by adulthood and remains stable throughout life. Most agree that behaviour will be determined by both personality and situation, and so the "expression" of personality can vary according to circumstances. This may be particularly important in the context of aging.

Describing personality

There are many different approaches to describing personality. Nomothetic approaches are divided into type (categorical) and trait (dimensional) approaches. The five-factor

The Old Age Psychiatry Handbook   Joanne Rodda, Niall Boyce, and Zuzana Walker
© 2008 John Wiley & Sons, Ltd

model is a well-known approach and describes personality using five dimensions (openness, conscientiousness, extraversion, agreeability, neuroticism).

Ideographic approaches to personality emphasise individuality and include psycho-analytical, humanistic and cognitive behavioural models. These approaches are more difficult to incorporate into scientific study.

Personality and age

Healthy adults

There is no clear answer to the question of whether or not personality changes with age. Several studies have demonstrated remarkable stability of personality factors with aging. Others have shown age-related changes in certain personality traits, including decreases in extraversion and conscientiousness and an increase in harm-avoidance.

It is possible that the apparent stability of personality with age relates to genetic factors and environmental stability. The changes reported in some studies may reflect adaptations to changing life-roles, medical co-morbidity and social circumstances. The issue is complex, as changes in behaviour do not necessarily reflect shifts in personality.

Aging does appear to have an impact on the prevalence and relative severity of personality disorders; this is discussed on page 127.

Personality change in the context of dementia

Dementia tends to increase self-centredness and decrease flexibility. Patients are often described as having "less" personality than before the dementia, for example less outgoing, less assertive, less conscientious.

Studies using the five-factor model of personality have shown changes in all factors in dementia. The most marked changes are decreased conscientiousness and extraversion and increased neuroticism.

It is important to recognise that changes in personality can occur even before the onset of dementia. In a patient presenting with personality change, dementia is an important differential diagnosis.

Frontotemporal dementia

Marked personality, affective and behavioural changes often precede the development of a generalised dementia syndrome in frontotemporal dementia. Disinhibition can lead to socially inappropriate, reckless and impulsive behaviour. A diagnosis of mood, psychotic or personality disorder may be given before the presence of frontotemporal dementia is recognised.

Dementia in patients with personality disorder

There may be an increase or decrease in the intensity of personality disorder in dementia, or the dementia may "neutralise" the personality disorder.

Personality changes in the context of medical illness

It has been suggested that chronic illness and an increased awareness of one's own mortality in old age leads to the exaggeration of life-long personality traits, contributing to maladaptive behavioural patterns in some patients.

Definition and classification of personality disorders

Both ICD-10 and DSM-IV describe personality disorders as persistent, pervasive and enduring patterns of inner experience and behaviour that begin in childhood or adolescence, continue into adulthood and are stable over time. These disorders manifest in cognitive, affective and behavioural patterns that deviate markedly from cultural norms and lead to distress or impairment.

Personality disorders are essentially clusters of symptoms and the validity of diagnostic criteria is often questioned. Validity in the elderly is even more unclear. The DSM-IV criteria for diagnosis of personality disorders are summarised in Table 7.1.

ICD-10

In ICD-10, the generic and specific criteria for personality disorders are very similar to DSM-IV. Differences in ICD-10 include:

1. Schizotypal disorder is coded under schizophrenia, schizotypal and delusional disorders.
2. Narcissistic personality disorder is not listed.
3. Dissocial personality disorder corresponds to antisocial personality disorder.
4. Anankastic personality corresponds to obsessive compulsive personality disorder.

Personality disorders in old age

Epidemiology

There are few epidemiological studies of personality disorder in old age. None of the instruments for assessment of personality disorder have been validated for use in elderly

Table 7.1 Summary of DSM-IV criteria for personality disorders

<table>
<tr><td colspan="2" align="center">**Generic criteria**</td></tr>
<tr><td colspan="2">Lasting pattern of behaviour and inner experience that markedly deviates from the patient's cultural norm, with roots in adolescence or early adulthood. Manifest in at least two of: affect, cognition, impulse control, interpersonal functioning. Pattern is fixed, affects many personal and social situations. Causes distress or impairs function. Not better explained by other psychiatric or medical diagnosis.</td></tr>
<tr><td colspan="2">Cluster A</td></tr>
<tr><td>**Paranoid**</td><td>Suspicious of others deceiving, exploiting or harming them. Reluctant to confide, bear persistent grudges, read hidden meanings and perceive innocent comments as personal attacks. Unwarranted suspicions of sexual infidelity of partner.</td></tr>
<tr><td>**Schizoid**</td><td>Do not want or like close relationships, prefer solitary activities. Little interest in sexual activity with another person. Enjoy few, if any, activities.</td></tr>
<tr><td>**Schizotypal**</td><td>Isolation and discomfort with social relationships. Lack close friends and confidants. Often odd beliefs, magical thinking, ideas of reference, unusual perceptions, paranoid/suspicious ideas and inappropriate affect. Anxiety in social situations is caused by paranoid fears.</td></tr>
<tr><td colspan="2">Cluster B</td></tr>
<tr><td>**Antisocial**</td><td>Irresponsible and often criminal behaviour begins in childhood/early adolescence. Characterised by aggression against people or animals, property destruction, lying, theft, violations of rules, disregard for rights of others, reckless or impulsive actions with notable lack of remorse.</td></tr>
<tr><td>**Borderline**</td><td>Unstable impulse control, interpersonal relationships, mood and self-image with frantic attempts to avoid abandonment. Self-mutilation, suicidal thoughts or threats, chronic feelings of emptiness, intense/inappropriate anger, brief paranoid ideas or stress-related dissociative symptoms.</td></tr>
<tr><td>**Histrionic**</td><td>Discomfort when not the centre of attention, inappropriately seductive or sexually provocative behaviour, shallow emotion with overly dramatic expression, use physical appearance to gain attention, vague speech, suggestibility, belief that relationships are more intimate than they are.</td></tr>
<tr><td>**Narcissitic**</td><td>Grandiosity, lack of empathy, arrogance and need for admiration. Exaggeration of own abilities/accomplishments. Preoccupation with fantasies of success, envy and uniqueness of own needs. Sense of entitlement with exploitation of others to achieve own goals.</td></tr>
<tr><td colspan="2">Cluster C</td></tr>
<tr><td>**Avoidant**</td><td>Hypersensitive to criticism. Avoid involvement with others for fear of criticism or rejection. Are convinced of being inadequate, inept or unappealing. New activities and relationships (especially intimate) are either avoided or fraught with fear of embarrassment, shame or ridicule.</td></tr>
<tr><td>**Dependent**</td><td>Desperately need approval of others. Convinced of a need to be taken care of and incapacity to function independently, fear abandonment. Need excessive advice and reassurance for everyday decisions. Behave submissively and avoid disagreement in order to gain and maintain nurture and support. If one relationship is lost, urgently seek replacement.</td></tr>
<tr><td>**Obsessive-compulsive**</td><td>Preoccupation with control, orderliness and perfection, often at the expense of task completion or to the extent that the purpose of the activity is lost. Tend to be workaholics, overly conscientious, inflexible and stingy with money. Often save worthless items, unable to throw them away.</td></tr>
</table>

patients and determining the presence of features since adolescence or early adulthood can be extremely difficult.

Estimates of prevalence of personality disorders in the elderly vary according to setting:

- Community: 2.8–13 %

- Psychiatric outpatients: 5–33 %

- Psychiatric inpatients: 7–61.5 %.

Diagnosis of personality disorder in late life

Although the features of personality disorder are present from early life, diagnosis is sometimes first made in old age. Possible explanations are:

- Changing roles and circumstances may reveal patterns of behaviour that were somehow "managed" or adaptive in earlier life.

- Personality disorder may be "eclipsed" by another psychiatric disorder (e.g. eating disorder, depression) in earlier life.

An individual with schizotypal disorder may live alone and go to work in a quiet environment with little need for interpersonal contact. His personality disorder may only be apparent when his increasing frailty in old age necessitates residential home care. Similarly, maladaptive personality traits may become apparent after the death of a spouse who was able to contain or "manage" them.

Changes in personality disorder with age

Cross-sectional studies of personality disorder in old age suggest that there is a lower prevalence of cluster B disorders and a higher prevalence of cluster C disorders. However, these studies are limited in what they can tell us about changes in personality disorder throughout life.

Borderline, antisocial, narcissistic and histrionic personality disorders have been described as "immature" personality disorders. Features of these disorders may be more evident in younger individuals and more moderate by mid-adulthood. Conversely, "mature" personality disorders (obsessive compulsive, paranoid, schizoid and schizotypal) may be more likely to remain stable for life. There is some evidence to support this. However, some suggest that features of borderline personality disorder are relatively dormant in middle life and re-emerge in old age.

Validity of personality disorder criteria in old age

It has been argued that personality disorder criteria are less relevant in the elderly because of physical limitations, changes in life roles and other ageing-related factors. For example:

• There may be fewer opportunities for recklessness/impulsivity

• Genuine disability may be interpreted as dependence

• Young adults need to separate from parents, form relationships and function in the workplace. The elderly face different challenges, for example retirement and losses in the form of bereavement or reduced independence.

Depression and personality disorders in old age

Rates of personality disorder in the elderly appear to be highest in people with depression and dysthymia, and have been reported to be as high as 31 % in this group. Cluster C traits, especially avoidant and dependent, are reported to be the most common.

This suggests that individuals with a personality disorder are more susceptible to depression in late life. One possible explanation is that personality disorder may stress adaptive capabilities to cope with life events. A further consideration is that the effects of a personality disorder in earlier life (e.g. divorce, employment instability) will often impact on support and other social factors in late life.

Personality disorder may affect the outcome of depression. In depressed elderly patients, it has been demonstrated that:

• Diagnosis of personality disorder is associated with failure of outpatient treatment.

• Avoidant and dependant traits are associated with lower functioning in activities of daily living.

• Paranoid, schizoid and narcissistic traits are associated with poorer social functioning.

A relationship between personality disorders and suicide in depression has not been demonstrated in studies of elderly people.

Anxiety and personality disorders in old age

In younger adults anxiety disorders are associated with high levels of neuroticism and cluster C traits of avoidance and dependence. This may also be the case in the elderly but has not been systematically studied.

Personality disorders and psychotic disorders in late life

Many people with late-onset schizophrenia will have had premorbid paranoid or schizoid personality disorders.

Management of personality disorder in old age

People with personality disorders can present particular challenges to management, both of the personality disorder itself and of co-morbid illness. There are higher rates of attrition and possibly litigiousness, and personality psychopathology may undermine the therapeutic alliance. These issues have not been investigated in the elderly but the picture may well be similar to that in younger adults.

Psychological treatments

General supportive therapy by a member of the team (e.g. support worker, social worker, community psychiatric nurse) may enable significant progress. There is very little research in specific therapies for personality disorder in the elderly. In younger adults various approaches are used although not all have evidence to support efficacy. These include:

- Dialectical behavioural therapy

- Interpersonal therapy

- Cognitive behavioural therapy

- Cognitive-analytic therapy

- Psychodynamic psychotherapy.

The most appropriate approach to management of personality disorders in the elderly will involve a consistent approach from all professionals involved in an individual's care. A psychologist or psychotherapist may be able to offer specific therapies. However, an equally important role may be to advise and support the team in the development and maintenance of a therapeutic relationship with the individual. Further information about psychological therapies is given on page 217.

Pharmacological treatment

Drug treatment of personality disorders in any age group is controversial. Limited evidence from studies in younger adults suggests that there might be some benefit from medication directed at specific symptoms rather than for a particular personality disorder, for example:

- Psychotic symptoms and hostility may respond to antipsychotic drugs.

- Depressive symptoms, suicidality, aggression and obsessionality may respond to antidepressants (particularly SSRIs).

- Mood stabilisers are sometimes used for affective fluctuations and aggression.

- Naltrexone has been used in deliberate self-harm (mutilation).

Pharmacotherapy may be effective in management of elderly patients with personality disorders but there have been no studies. Given the lack of an evidence base and the susceptibility of elderly people to adverse drug reactions, drug treatment may be best reserved for management of co-morbid psychiatric illness.

Further reading

Abrams RC and Bromberg CE (2006) Personality disorders in the elderly: a flagging field of enquiry *Int J Geriat Psychiat* 21: 1013–1017.

Bateman AW and Tyrer P (2004) Psychological treatment of personality disorders *Adv Psychiat Treat* 10: 378–388.

Lautenschlager NT and Forstl H (2007) Personality change in old age *Curr Opin Psychiat* 20: 62–66.

Segal DL, Coolridge FL and Rosowsky E (2006) *Personality Disorders and Older Adults. Diagnosis, Assessment and Treatment* New York, John Wiley & Sons.

Seidlitz L (2001) Personality factors in mental disorders of later life *Am J Geriat Psychiat* 9: 8–21.

Tyrer P and Bateman AW (2004) Drug treatment for personality disorders *Adv Psychiat Treat* 10: 389–398.

8

Alcohol

Alcohol misuse in the elderly is an important and often overlooked issue. Studies have demonstrated significant rates of potentially harmful drinking and alcohol dependence in old age. Older people are more susceptible to the harmful effects of alcohol, mainly due to physiological changes, exacerbation of chronic illness and interaction with prescribed medication. There is evidence that the elderly respond as well as if not better than younger people to interventions aimed at reducing alcohol intake.

Current guidelines for alcohol consumption

An individual's alcohol consumption does not have to increase to be a problem as they grow older. Age-related changes in body composition and metabolism mean that older people are more sensitive to the effects of alcohol. What may seem like a reasonable weekly intake in a younger adult may be excessive as they move into old age. Older people are also more likely to have medical illnesses and take medication that may interact adversely with alcohol.

The Old Age Psychiatry Handbook   Joanne Rodda, Niall Boyce, and Zuzana Walker
© 2008 John Wiley & Sons, Ltd

Table 8.1 Alcohol units and standard drinks

			Approximate equivalents		
Country	Basic unit	Alcohol	Beer	Wine	Spirits
UK	Unit	8 g	250 ml	85 ml	25 ml
USA	Standard drink	13 g	360 ml	150 ml	45 ml

The UK Department of Health does not currently make specific recommendations for safe drinking in the elderly. General advice is to consume no more than three to four units per day for men and two to three units per day for women. Recommendations for the elderly would need to be lower than this.

The National Institute on Alcohol Abuse and Alcoholism (NIAAA, USA) recommend that people over the age of 65 do not consume more than one standard drink per day. Alcohol units and "standard drinks" are summarised in Table 8.1.

Definitions

Abstinence

There is no consumption of alcohol at all (more specifically for one year).

Low risk/moderate consumption

Alcohol consumption within recommended limits and that does not have adverse consequences.

Problem drinking/at risk use

Drinking at a level that results in/is likely to result in adverse medical, psychological or social consequences but dependence has not been reached. ICD-10 uses the term "harmful use" to describe consumption of a substance that results in clear physical or psychological harm without dependence.

Dependence

The alcohol dependence syndrome was initially characterised by Edwards and Gross in 1976. ICD-10 and DSM-IV criteria for depression are based on this definition. Features of dependence are:

- Strong desire or compulsion to drink

- Loss of control of drinking in terms of onset, duration and amount

- Withdrawal symptoms if alcohol is not consumed

- Tolerance to the effects of alcohol

- Preoccupation with alcohol at expense of other aspects of life

- Much time spent obtaining, drinking and recovering from the effects of alcohol

- Persistent drinking despite evidence of harmful consequences

- Rapid reinstatement of the syndrome after a period of abstinence.

Epidemiology

Approximately two thirds of alcohol dependent elderly individuals will have had onset in earlier life. Consumption of alcohol usually reduces with age and 50–60 % of elderly people are abstinent. However, for some people, drinking will increase in old age, for example as a result of unstructured or excess free time, bereavements or memory problems.

Estimates of the prevalence of problem drinking and alcohol dependence vary according to definitions and the population studied. Around 10–15 % of over 65s in the community consume more than the recommended amount of alcohol. The one-year community prevalence rate for alcohol abuse and dependence in the elderly is estimated at 2.75 % for men and 0.51 % for women. In certain ethnic minority groups such as the elderly Asian population alcohol use is very uncommon.

Detection and screening

Excess alcohol consumption in the elderly often goes undetected. This may be in part because healthcare professionals do not expect to find problem drinking in this group. In addition, problems at work or with the police often lead to the presentation of alcohol-related disorders in younger adults and this is much less likely to happen in the elderly.

An accurate alcohol history is an important part of any psychiatric assessment and it is good practice to routinely screen for problem drinking. The CAGE questionnaire (Box 8.1) is widely used in the elderly. The Short Michigan Alcohol Screening Test – Geriatric (SMAST-G, Box 8.2) has been specifically developed for use in elderly populations. The AUDIT questionnaire asks more specific questions about frequency and quantities consumed.

Box 8.1   CAGE questionnaire

Have you ever felt you should **C**ut down on your drinking?

Has anyone ever **A**nnoyed you by criticising your drinking?

Have you ever felt **G**uilty about your drinking?

Have you ever had a drink early in the morning as an **E**ye-opener?

Two or more questions answered yes is indicative of problem drinking

---

Box 8.2   Short Michigan Alcohol Screening Test – Geriatric (SMAST-G*)

1. When talking with others do you ever underestimate how much you actually drink?

2. After a few drinks, have you sometimes not eaten or been able to skip a meal because you're not hungry?

3. Does having a few drinks help decrease your shakiness or tremors?

4. Does alcohol sometimes make it hard for you to remember parts of the day or night?

5. Do you usually take a drink to relax or calm your nerves?

6. Do you drink to take your mind off problems?

7. Have you ever increased your drinking after experiencing a loss in your life?

8. Has a doctor or a nurse ever said they were worried or concerned about your drinking?

9. Have you ever made rules to manage your drinking?

10. When you feel lonely, does a drink help?

Three or more questions answered yes is indicative of problem drinking

*The SMAST-G Questionnaire is reproduced by permission of the University of Michigan Alcohol Research Center.

Blood tests

There are no specific blood tests that are sensitive enough for use in screening for alcohol disorders. However, routine blood tests performed for another reason sometimes suggest the possibility of an alcohol problem:

- Elevated γ-GT (less often elevated ALT or AST)

- Macrocytic anaemia

- Low platelets

- Elevated cholesterol.

Consequences

Positive effects

There is limited evidence that moderate alcohol consumption has beneficial effects related to cardiovascular and dementia risk. However, most of these studies were in middle-aged men and the risk:benefit ratio in elderly people may be different.

Medical complications

Older people are more susceptible and less resilient than younger adults to the medical complications of alcohol misuse (Table 8.2), including the development of nutritional deficiencies. Elderly people who develop cirrhosis are more likely than younger adults to die within one year of diagnosis.

Drug interactions

Alcohol markedly increases the risk of adverse drug reactions. There are adverse interactions with most psychiatric drugs. The effects of alcohol on drug metabolism can lead to dangerous interactions with warfarin and digoxin.

Anxiety and depression

Symptoms of anxiety and depression are common in alcohol abuse and often meet criteria for diagnosis of a specific disorder. It is often difficult to establish cause and effect.

Table 8.2 Complications of alcohol misuse

Hepatic	Alcoholic liver disease
	– fatty change
	– alcoholic hepatitis
	– cirrhosis
	Hepatocellular carcinoma
Gastrointestinal	Haematemesis caused by:
	– gastritis/peptic ulceration
	– oesophageal varices
	– Mallory-Weiss tears
	Pancreatitis
	Chronic diarrhoea
Cardiovascular	Hypertension
	Atrial fibrillation and other arrhythmias
	Cerebrovascular accident
	Dilated cardiomyopathy
Neurological	Wernicke-Korsakoff syndrome
	Peripheral neuropathy
	Alcoholic myopathy
	Cerebellar degeneration
	Optic atrophy
	Central pontine myelinosis
Musculoskeletal	Gout
	Osteoporosis
Psychiatric	Anxiety/depression
	Sleep disturbances
	Alcoholic hallucinosis
	Alcohol-related cognitive impairment and dementia
Withdrawal	Withdrawal symptoms, including seizures
	Delirium tremens
Other	Drug interactions
	Falls
	Impairment of driving skills
	Loss of social support networks

Suicide

The lifetime risk of suicide in those with alcohol dependence is estimated at 7 %. In a study of suicides in adults over the age of 65, alcohol misuse or dependence was present in 35 % of men and 18 % of women.

Important risk factors for suicide in the context of alcohol problems are:

- Age over 50

- Psychiatric co-morbidity, especially depression

- Medical co-morbidity

- Repeated failed attempts at abstinence.

Other risk factors and issues relating to suicide are discussed on page 76.

Alcoholic hallucinosis

Alcoholic hallucinosis is a rare complication of prolonged heavy alcohol use. Elderly people whose alcohol dependence began in younger adulthood are therefore at the highest risk. Hallucinations are almost always auditory and occur in clear consciousness whilst sober. In the vast majority the problem responds to antipsychotic medication and resolves on cessation of drinking. A small proportion will go on to develop a schizophrenia-like illness.

Cognitive impairment

Cognitive deficits are apparent in the majority of heavy drinkers whilst sober, particularly impairment of memory and executive function. These deficits may have a more significant impact on functioning in elderly people with reduced cognitive reserve.

Alcoholic dementia (page 51) occurs in the context of prolonged severe alcohol abuse. It is believed to be caused by the direct neurotoxic effects of alcohol. The dementia may be partially reversible on abstinence.

Structural changes are found on CT and MRI in chronic alcohol abuse:

- Loss of grey matter

- Enlargement of ventricles

- Thinning of corpus callosum.

These changes correlate poorly with the degree of cognitive deficit and may be partially reversible on abstinence. Women are more susceptible than men.

Wernicke-Korsakoff syndrome

Wernicke encephalopathy

Alcohol affects the absorption and activation of thiamine. Severe thiamine deficiency results in acute presentation with:

- Acute confusional state

- Opthalmoplegia

- Pupillary abnormalities

- Nystagmus

- Ataxia.

Management involves parenteral vitamin replacement and supportive therapy, including treatment of alcohol withdrawal (see below). It is essential that thiamine replacement is given before carbohydrate replacement. Untreated, the acute phase lasts for approximately two weeks; 20 % will die and 75 % will develop Korsakoff's psychosis.

Korsakoff psychosis

Korsakoff psychosis in an amnestic syndrome that is caused by thiamine deficiency. It usually occurs in the context of alcohol abuse and may follow untreated Wernicke encephalopathy. Features are:

- Inability to form new memories

- Variable retrograde amnesia

- Intact working and procedural memory.

Prognosis is poor although a minority may improve on abstinence. Overall 25 % require long-term residential care; this figure will be higher if the syndrome develops in old age.

Social consequences

Social consequences of alcohol problems include:

• Damage to relationships with family and friends

• Breakdown of social networks

• Impairment of driving skills and increased road traffic accidents.

If the patient continues to drive against advice and/or refuses to inform the DVLA of a diagnosis of alcohol misuse or dependence then it is the duty of the doctor responsible for their care to do so (page 238).

Management

Psychosocial interventions

Brief interventions range from unstructured counselling to short courses of structured therapy. Studies have shown that as little as one brief counselling session can be effective in reducing alcohol consumption in elderly problem drinkers in primary care.

Elderly people with alcohol dependence benefit as much as if not more than young adults from *group therapy*, either in residential or outpatient settings. More benefit is gained from age-specific rather than mixed-age groups. Access to this type of service is often limited.

Agencies such as *Alcoholics Anonymous* (http://www.alcoholics-anonymous.org.uk) also provide services for older adults, but may not run age-specific groups.

Pharmacological treatment

Pharmacological therapy may be used in some patients as an adjunct to psychosocial interventions.

Naltrexone is an opiate antagonist that is believed to reduce the reinforcing effects of alcohol. It may help to maintain abstinence or reduced consumption of alcohol. There are limited studies in the elderly but current evidence supports good tolerability and reduced relapse rates.

Acamprosate is used in younger adults to reduce craving for alcohol. It is only suitable for individuals who wish to achieve and maintain abstinence. There are no studies of its use in the elderly.

Disulfiram has an unpleasant interaction with alcohol that deters individuals from impulsive drinking. It is generally avoided in the elderly.

Detoxification and withdrawal

Acute alcohol withdrawal

Alcohol-dependent individuals admitted to hospital are at risk of acute withdrawal (Box 8.3). Information about alcohol consumption may not be volunteered and so is an important part of the history. Alcohol consumption may also be involuntarily limited during respite care or a move to a residential home, resulting in withdrawal symptoms.

Box 8.3   Clinical features of alcohol withdrawal

Anxiety

Agitation

Sweating

Tachycardia

Coarse tremor

Nausea and vomiting

Insomnia

Seizures

Management involves a reducing regime of a benzodiazepine, usually diazepam or chlordiazepoxide:

- Duration of treatment is usually five to seven days

- Dose will depend on the individual

- The elderly are generally very susceptible to the effects of benzodiazepines but alcohol increases tolerance

- There is no evidence that longer duration of withdrawal treatment is required in the elderly.

In addition, vitamin replacement is essential:

- Parenteral vitamin B1 (Pabrinex: two ampoules b.d. for three days)

- Vitamin replacement must be given before carbohydrate replacement to avoid precipitation of Wernicke encephalopathy.

Delirium tremens

Delirium tremens (Box 8.4) is a life-threatening condition resulting from acute alcohol withdrawal:

- It develops 1–7 days after the last drink.

- Peak is at 2–3 days.

- Overall mortality is 5–10 %, this is likely to be higher in the elderly.

- Outcome is worst in unexpected/undetected cases.

- Patients need urgent transfer to medical ward/intensive care (ITU).

Box 8.4 Clinical features of delirium tremens

Features of uncomplicated alcohol withdrawal plus:

−acute confusional state

−marked agitation

−visual, auditory and tactile hallucinations (Lilliputian, formication)

−paranoid delusions

−sudden cardiovascular collapse

Further reading

Oslin W (2004) Late-life alcoholism. Issues relevant to the geriatric psychiatrist *Am J Geriat Psychiat* 12: 571–583.

Oslin W (2005) Evidence based treatment of geriatric substance abuse *Psychiat Clin N Am* 28: 897–911.

Thomson AD and Marshall EJ (2006) The natural history and pathophysiology of Wernicke's Encephalopathy and Korsakoff's psychosis *Alcohol Alcoholism* 41: 151–158

Whelan G (2003) Alcohol: a much neglected risk factor in elderly mental disorders *Curr Opin Psychiat* 16: 609–614.

9
Insomnia

One of the most common problems experienced by older adults is difficulty sleeping. It is estimated that 40 % of elderly people experience insomnia, but despite this high prevalence it is often under-treated. Pharmacological management is generally unsatisfactory. However, an understanding of sleep architecture and the causes of insomnia in the elderly can enable implementation of effective non-pharmacological approaches.

Sleep architecture

Sleep architecture describes the makeup of a night's sleep in terms of several distinct types of sleep (Table 9.1). The two main types of sleep, REM and non-REM, alternate throughout the night. Non-REM sleep is further divided into four stages. Sleep is entered through stage 1 sleep. Stages 3 and 4 (slow wave sleep) are believed to be the most restorative. Each type of sleep has a distinct EEG pattern.

The Old Age Psychiatry Handbook   Joanne Rodda, Niall Boyce, and Zuzana Walker
© 2008 John Wiley & Sons, Ltd

Table 9.1   Normal sleep architecture

Non-REM sleep	Stage 1	Light sleep	Predominates in second third of night
	Stage 2		
	Stage 3	Deep/slow wave sleep	Predominates in first third of night
	Stage 4		
REM sleep	Approximately five discrete episodes throughout night		
	Predominates in last third of night		

With aging, there are a number of changes in sleep architecture (Box 9.1). Overall, elderly people have a decreased quantity and quality of sleep and reduced sleep efficiency (ratio of time spent in bed to time actually asleep).

Box 9.1   Changes in sleep architecture with age

Total sleep time reduced due to:

– increased time to initiation of sleep

– increased frequency of awakenings

– earlier waking

Increased percentage of light sleep

Reduced percentage of slow wave (deep) sleep

Reduced REM sleep

– increased REM latency

– reduced percentage of REM sleep

Increased frequency of daytime napping

Fragmentation of sleep cycle

Reduced overall sleep quality and efficiency

Circadian rhythm

Circadian rhythms are the biological rhythms of the body, including the sleep–wake cycle. Circadian rhythm becomes less synchronised with age and can result in disruption of sleeping patterns. Exposure to light as an external cue during the day can help to normalise circadian rhythm.

Insomnia and consequences in the elderly

Insomnia is the subjective experience of insufficient or inadequate sleep and is the most common sleep complaint in the elderly. It is associated with:

* Decreased memory and concentration

* General cognitive impairment

* Falls

* Increased mortality.

Causes of insomnia

Although changes in sleep architecture are a normal part of aging, these changes do not on their own account for the high prevalence of insomnia in the elderly.

Transient (lasting for few nights) and *acute* (lasting for no more than four weeks) insomnia are usually caused by a brief stressor or disruption, for example acute illness, environmental changes or jet lag.

Chronic insomnia is insomnia lasting for more than four weeks. Causes include:

* *Primary sleep disorders*, e.g. circadian rhythm disorders, sleep apnoea and REM sleep behaviour disorder (see page 48).

* *Physical illnesses* causing pain, discomfort, breathlessness or necessitating regular waking (e.g. nocturia in prostatic disease).

* Most *psychiatric illnesses*.

* *Dementia*, which can significantly affect sleep architecture and reverse circadian rhythm. Sleep changes in people with dementia are common and tend to be more severe than in those without.

- Prescribed and over the counter *drugs*.

- *Nicotine* and *caffeine* (central nervous system stimulants).

- *Alcohol*.

- *Environmental* factors, e.g. noise, temperature, uncomfortable bed.

- *Behavioural* factors, e.g. daytime napping, eating a meal before bed.

Assessment of a patient with insomnia

Establishing the *24-hour sleep pattern* (Box 9.2) will help diagnosis of insomnia and may help to identify a cause. The easiest way to do this is by using a two-week *sleep diary* although this may be difficult for some patients, for example those with dementia.

Box 9.2   Establishing a 24-hour sleep pattern

Duration of symptoms

Usual bed time

Time taken to fall asleep

Usual waking time

Usual getting-up time

Number of awakenings

Daytime sleep

Total quantity of sleep

Particularly important information from the history of a patient presenting with insomnia is:

- Duration of the problem

- 24-hour sleep pattern

- Physical illness

- Medication

- Presence of other causes listed above

- History from bed partner (e.g. sleepwalking, snoring, jerking)

- Impact of insomnia.

More advanced methods of assessment include video recording of sleep and polysomnography using EEG and EMG but these are rarely indicated.

Non-pharmacological management

Non-pharmacological strategies (Table 9.2) should always be first line in the management of insomnia. In many cases, it will be necessary to address physical illness or medication issues that are causing or contributing to the insomnia.

Sleep hygiene measures (Table 9.3) are directed at optimising behaviours and environmental conditions that favour sleep, and can be helpful for all patients with insomnia. Insomnia is often a problem in patients with dementia, and helping carers to implement good sleep hygiene practices for the patient can have positive results.

Pharmacological management

The benefits of hypnotic drugs must be balanced against the risks of tolerance, dependence and falls in the elderly.

Occasionally it is justified to prescribe a hypnotic drug for a brief period, but longer periods of prescribing can lead to an exacerbation of the problem because of rebound

Table 9.2 Non-pharmacological management of insomnia

Sleep hygiene	Basic measures aimed at sleep environment and behaviours that affect sleep.
Sleep restriction	Restricting time in bed to the number of hours asleep, increasing time in bed as sleep efficiency increases.
Cognitive therapy	Addresses maladaptive cognitions related to sleep.
Relaxation techniques	Aims to reduce the level of anxiety and arousal associated with insomnia.

Table 9.3 Principles of sleep hygiene

Environment	Behaviours to encourage
Comfortable	Regular schedule of bed time and getting up
Familiar	Regular exercise
Quiet	Maximise light exposure during day
Dark	Go to bed only when tired

Behaviours to avoid
Use of caffeine, nicotine or alcohol late in day
Daytime naps, especially after 2 pm
Heavy meals near bed time
Exercise near bed time
Drinking a lot of fluids in the evening
Talking or thinking about worries near bed time

insomnia when the drug is stopped. Principles of drug treatment of insomnia in the elderly are:

- Short-term prescribing (two to four weeks)

- Use lowest possible dose

- Use medications with short half-lives (Table 10.42)

- Use intermittent dosing (e.g. two to four times per week)

- Gradual withdrawal of medication to avoid rebound insomnia.

The drugs most commonly used in the management of insomnia are the benzodiazepines and the "Z" drugs (zopiclone, zolpidem, zaleplon). The properties of these drugs and their effects on sleep are covered on page 198. Some claim that the shorter half-lives of the "Z" drugs, particularly zaleplon, make them safer to use in the elderly. However, this is not clear and the level of risk may be similar to the benzodiazepines.

Further reading

Ancoli-Israel A and Ayalon L (2006) Diagnosis and treatment of sleep disorders in older adults *Am J Geriat Psychiat* 14: 95–103.
Kamel NS and Kammack JK (2006) Insomnia in the elderly: cause, approach and treatment *Am J Med* 119: 463–469.

10

Psychopharmacology

Principles of drug treatment in old age psychiatry

There are a number of factors to consider when prescribing medication for the elderly. Older people are more sensitive to adverse drug reactions, are more likely to have co-morbid illness and are frequently prescribed multiple medications. There may also be difficulties with adherence. Many of the risks associated with drug treatment in old age can be minimised by adhering to a few basic principles (Box 10.1).

The Old Age Psychiatry Handbook   Joanne Rodda, Niall Boyce, and Zuzana Walker
© 2008 John Wiley & Sons, Ltd

Box 10.1　Basic principles of prescribing for older people

Minimise the number of drugs

Use simple medication regimes

Avoid drugs associated with adverse reactions in the elderly

Start at low doses, with titration if necessary

Review medication regularly

Use adherence aids or medication supervision where necessary

Ensure good communication between professionals

This chapter focuses on the rationale behind these principles. Each section covers either a specific aspect of prescribing or important information about a specific class of drugs.

Evidence base

Most trials of psychiatric drugs exclude older people and evidence from studies of young adults is often extrapolated for older patients. Specific studies of older people are often small and may exclude important groups, for example those with co-morbid illness or cognitive impairment. With the increasing number of elderly patients, the evidence base will continue to grow and provide clearer information upon which to base decisions. This section will attempt to describe the best practice based on currently available evidence.

Adherence

Medication only works when it is taken, and adherence is a subject relevant to all areas of medicine. Whilst the incidence of cognitive impairment, polypharmacy and adverse drug reactions increases with age, studies have not been consistent in demonstrating a relationship between age and adherence. Certain factors that may impair adherence occur less frequently in the elderly, for example chaotic lifestyle or substance misuse. The issues relevant to medication adherence in old age psychiatry are outlined below.

Factors relating to the illness

Severity of psychosis is associated with poor adherence with medication. There may be apathy in schizophrenia or depression, and insight into the need for treatment can be

Table 10.1   Factors relating to the illness and the patient that may affect
adherence

Illness factors	Patient factors
Severity of the illness	Attitudes towards medication and health professionals
Insight	Educational level
Apathy	Alcohol misuse
Cognitive impairment	Impaired dexterity
Delusions	Visual impairment
	Swallowing problems
	Co-administration of other medication

impaired in any mental illness. Studies have demonstrated improvements in adherence
from cognitive behavioural therapy combined with psychoeducation and also from family
therapy.

In dementia, people may simply forget to take their tablets and a dosette box can be
helpful. The patient (or if necessary a relative or friend) puts the tablets into a box with
separate sections according to time and day of the week. Pharmacies can also fill in dosette
boxes or make up blister packs. Some people with dementia will require supervision
with medication from a relative or a carer. Paid carers are allowed to supervise but not
dispense medication, and so a pre-filled dosette box or blister pack is necessary in this
situation.

Paradoxically, people with severe dementia have better adherence than those with
moderate dementia because they are likely to receive more intensive supervision.

Factors relating to the patient

Problems caused by physical disabilities can be relatively easy to address if they are
recognised:

- Non-childproof containers for patients with poor dexterity

- Use of dosette boxes

- Liquid medication if it is easier for the patient to swallow, however it can be more
  difficult to measure out the correct dose

- Assistance from a relative or carer when taking medication.

When multiple medications are prescribed, adherence is often reduced because of
the increased incidence of side effects and/or complicated medication regimes. Again,

minimising the number of tablets, simplifying the regime (e.g. once daily dosing) and using dosette boxes or blister packs can help.

There is also a strong positive association between alcohol misuse and non-adherence. This issue is more difficult to address but it is important to bear in mind if there are concerns about adherence.

Factors relating to the drug

People are less likely to take a drug if they feel that it is not working, causes side effects or has to be taken very frequently. Explanation of the effects of the drug, delays in onset of action and why there is a need for maintenance treatment even in the absence of symptoms can improve adherence. Regular reviews of medication enable any issues related to side effects, poor efficacy and interactions to be addressed.

Box 10.2   Factors relating to the drug that may affect adherence

Efficacy

Delayed onset of action

Side effects

Frequency of doses

Drug interactions

Requirement of maintenance treatment

Factors relating to the doctor

The quality of the doctor-patient relationship has been shown to affect adherence. Fully informing patients about the rationale for the medication and its risks and benefits does not reduce adherence and involving the patient in decision making in this way may improve the doctor-patient relationship.

Summary

Many of the factors that affect adherence in general medicine and psychiatry are also important in the elderly, as well as issues that are specific for this population. Simple interventions can be successful in improving adherence (Box 10.3).

Box 10.3   Improving adherence – summary

Provide clear information about risks and benefits of medication

Involve patient in decision making

Implement simple medication regimes

Minimise side effects

— choose drugs with good side effect profiles

— use lowest possible dose

Regularly review medication

Where indicated ensure:

— non-childproof containers

— dosette boxes or individual blister packs

— supervision of medication

— specific psychological therapies aimed at improving adherence

Pharmacokinetics and pharmacodynamics

Pharmacokinetic changes associated with ageing

Pharmacokinetics describes the processes by which the body deals with a drug and can be summarised in terms of:

- Absorption

- Distribution

- Metabolism

- Elimination.

In addition to changes associated with age, there is also an increase in inter-individual variability of pharmacokinetic profiles. Two people in their eighties are more likely to have a different plasma concentration of a drug after being given the same dose than are two individuals in their thirties.

Intestinal absorption

Despite the changes in the intestinal wall that come with age, the total amount of drug absorbed is generally not affected. The process may be slowed by the reduction in splanchnic blood flow. Drug action may therefore be delayed, which can be of significance if the medication is given to act at a specific time (e.g. hypnotics and analgesics). This will be exacerbated by prescribing medications with anticholinergic side effects because of the resulting reduction in intestinal motility.

In a few cases where drugs are transported across the intestinal wall by active transport systems (for example B vitamins, iron) absorption may be slowed with age.

Body water and body fat

Box 10.4   Volume of distribution

The volume of distribution refers to the amount of a drug distributed throughout the body compared to the amount of drug in the plasma.

When given as a figure it refers to the total volume that the body would have to be if the amount of drug given was distributed at the same concentration as in the plasma.

The volume of distribution is *high* if there is a low concentration of drug in the plasma compared to the rest of the body.

The volume of distribution is *low* if there is a high concentration of drug in the plasma compared to the rest of the body.

In older people there is a lower proportion of body water. Total body water content falls by 10–19 % each year until the age of about 80, resulting in a decreased volume of distribution (Box 10.4) for water-soluble drugs such as lithium and aspirin.

In contrast to total body water, the percentage of body fat increases with age. Fat-soluble drugs (for example benzodiazepines, most antipsychotics and antidepressants) therefore have an increased volume of distribution in older people.

Plasma protein binding

Plasma protein binding of drugs reduces with age. Drugs that are normally highly protein-bound (e.g. sodium valproate, olanzapine and sertraline) may therefore have higher free levels in the elderly. These changes are not usually of clinical relevance in healthy older people. In situations where there is a significant reduction in albumin levels (e.g. malnutrition and physical illness) there may be an increase in free drug levels that needs to be taken into consideration.

Hepatic drug metabolism

Most psychotropic drugs are extensively metabolised by the liver, with the exception of sulpiride, amisulpiride and lithium. In old age, physiological changes, reduced liver mass and decreased blood flow may inhibit the delivery of a drug to hepatocytes. As a result there is often a decline in the elimination of psychotropic drugs. This may be particularly true of drugs that are metabolised by the cytochrome P450 system (page 161) and that normally have a high degree of first pass metabolism.

Use of drugs in hepatic impairment. Hepatic function generally declines in older people and the likelihood of more significant impairment also increases. Some drugs are contraindicated in hepatic impairment and others can be used with varying degrees of caution (Table 10.2). Most drugs that are not contraindicated will need some dose adjustment, especially with more severe impairment, and the half-life of many drugs will be increased. In all cases, it is important to refer to prescribing guidelines. Risks have to be balanced against benefits and medication needs to be carefully monitored and reviewed.

Table 10.2 Drugs to avoid and safer options for prescribing in patients with hepatic impairment

Group	Drugs to avoid	Safer options
Antidepressants	Tricyclics MAOIs Duloxetine	Citalopram[*] Paroxetine[*]
Antipsychotics	Phenothiazines (chlorpromazine, fluphenazine, levomepromazine)	Sulpiride Amisulpiride Haloperidol[*]
Mood stabilisers	Lamotrigine Valproate	Lithium
Anxiolytics and hypnotics	Caution with all sedatives, risk of precipitating hepatic encephalopathy	Lorazepam[**] Oxazepam[**] Temazepam[**] Zopiclone[**]

[*]Relatively safe but dose reduction/low starting dose recommended
[**]Use low doses with caution; sedation may precipitate hepatic encephalopathy
Sources: Maudsley Prescribing Guidelines 2007, British National Formulary September 2007

Renal drug elimination

The reduction in elimination of drugs by the kidney is the most significant pharmacokinetic change associated with old age. Elderly people can be assumed to have mild renal impairment, although serum creatinine is often not elevated because of reduced muscle mass. There is decreased:

- Renal blood flow

- Glomerular filtration rate

- Tubular secretion.

Some drugs are excreted unaltered by the kidneys whilst others undergo significant metabolism in the liver, and their metabolites (which may be active or inactive) are excreted by the kidneys. A reduction in renal elimination can lead to accumulation of the unaltered drug or its metabolites and so the safest drugs to use are those that undergo metabolism to inactive metabolites in the liver (Table 10.3).

Use of drugs in renal impairment   The presence of renal impairment necessitates extra care in prescribing. As with hepatic impairment, some drugs are contraindicated whilst others can be used with caution. Dose reductions are usually necessary and it is important to refer to prescribing guidelines.

Table 10.3   Drugs to avoid and safer options for prescribing in patients with renal impairment

Group	Drugs to avoid	Safer options
Antidepressants	Lofepramine	Citalopram Sertraline
Antipsychotics	Amisulpiride Sulpiride	Olanzapine Haloperidol
Mood stabilisers	Lithium	Valproate Carbamazepine Lamotrigine*
Anxiolytics and hypnotics	Sedation more likely in patients with renal impairment; caution needed with all anxiolytics and hypnotics	Lorazepam* Zopiclone*

*Relatively safe but dose reduction necessary. Caution is required with all drugs in renal impairment especially when more severe
Sources: Maudsley Prescribing Guidelines 2007, British National Formulary September 2007

Pharmacodynamic changes associated with ageing

The effect of a drug once it reaches its target receptor is dependent on:

• The number and properties of the receptor

• The response of the cell to receptor occupation

• Counter-regulation by homeostatic mechanisms to maintain a safe equilibrium.

Receptor changes

There are many changes in receptor quantity and activation that mean that older people can be more sensitive to both the beneficial and the adverse effects of drugs. This often means that lower doses of a drug are needed to achieve the desired effect or that significant side effects occur at therapeutic doses. Age-influenced receptor changes that are particularly relevant to old age psychiatry include:

• The reduction in dopamine receptor and dopamine transporter levels leads to increased sensitivity to dopaminergic blockade (e.g. increased incidence of extrapyramidal side effects of antipsychotic drugs).

• Reduced numbers of acetylcholine receptors cause increased sensitivity to anticholinergic effects of drugs.

• Changes in the $GABA_A$-benzodiazepine receptor complex cause increased sensitivity to the effects of benzodiazepines.

• Changes in α-1 adrenoreceptors lead to an increased risk of postural hypotension (see below).

• Changes in β-adrenergic receptors increase susceptibility to cardiac side effects of drugs.

• Changes in signal transduction pathways may be relevant but little is yet known about this area.

Homeostatic mechanisms

The general decline in homeostatic regulatory mechanisms with ageing renders older people more susceptible to the effects of drugs that challenge the physiological equilibrium.

Table 10.4 Impaired homeostatic responses in the elderly

Impaired homeostatic response	Potential outcome
Impaired balance response	Falls
Delayed postural circulatory response	Falls and syncope
Poor thermoregulation	Hypo- and hyper-thermia
Lack of thirst	Dehydration
Impaired laryngeal reflexes	Choking and aspiration

The impact of relatively minor side effects can be magnified in the context of the lack of homeostatic reserve outlined in Table 10.4. A mild sedative side effect of a drug may not be a problem in a young adult, but the same level of sedation in an 80 year old can result in falls, aspiration or dehydration. People with reduced cognitive reserve are also more susceptible to confusion.

The elderly are much more vulnerable to the effects of drugs that reduce arterial blood pressure. Psychiatric drugs with hypotensive side effects (for example antipsychotics and benzodiazepines) are more likely to cause postural hypotension, syncope and falls in older people.

Summary

The overall impact of ageing on the effects of a drug is determined by the balance of the age-related changes affecting the way that the body handles and responds to drugs. It is clearly not possible to predict the exact response of a patient to a specific drug at a given dose, but taking into account the basic principles of age-associated pharmacokinetic and pharmacodynamic changes enables safer and more rational prescribing.

Adverse drug reactions and interactions

Older people are far more susceptible than the young to both adverse drug reactions (ADRs) and interactions. Frail elderly people and nursing home residents are particularly vulnerable.

Several factors contribute to the increased risk of ADRs and interactions in the elderly:

- Age-related pharmacokinetic changes (page 153):

  - reduction in renal elimination

  - reduction in hepatic metabolism

  - reduction in plasma binding of drugs increases free drug levels.

- Age related pharmacodynamic changes (page 157).

- Increased likelihood of co-morbid illness.

- Increased number of drugs prescribed (polypharmacy).

Co-morbidity

Older people have an increased risk of physical illness, which can have a marked effect on the actions and safety of any drug. As above, considerations include pharmacokinetic and pharmacodynamic factors (see Table 10.5 for examples) and the increased likelihood of polypharmacy.

Polypharmacy

Polypharmacy is a major issue in the elderly. In the US the average older person takes at least three prescribed medications, with 11 % of the elderly taking more than ten medications and the average nursing home resident taking seven. Old people with depression take more medications than those without. The number of adverse drug reactions increases exponentially with the number of medications.

A major difficulty in managing polypharmacy is that there is often more than one doctor prescribing for the same patient. Good communication between professionals with regular reviews of medication is therefore essential.

Adverse drug reactions

ADRs are either dose related or idiosyncratic and the elderly are more susceptible to both types for the reasons highlighted above. Up to 20 % of hospital admissions in the

Table 10.5 Examples of pharmacokinetic and pharmacodynamic effects of illness on drug handling and actions

Mechanism	Example
Pharmacokinetic	Reduced renal elimination of drugs in diabetic nephropathy and heart failure
	Reduced protein binding of drugs in cachexia secondary to chronic illness
	Reduced absorption of drugs following intestinal resection
Pharmacodynamic	Exacerbation of hypertension by venlafaxine
	Tricyclic antidepressants can exacerbate arrhythmias
	SSRIs can increase risk of gastrointestinal bleeding

Table 10.6 Important side effects mediated by antagonism at muscarinic acetylcholine, α_1 adrenergic and histamine (H$_1$) receptors

Anticholinergic (muscarinic)	Antiadrenergic (α_1)	Antihistaminic (H$_1$)
Confusion	Orthostatic hypotension	Sedation
Hallucinations	– dizziness	Weight gain
Sedation	– falls	
Blurred vision		
Dry mouth	Sexual dysfunction	
Urinary retention		
Constipation		

elderly are caused by ADRs, of which 80 % are dose related and therefore to some extent predictable based on the pharmacological properties of the drugs.

Many of the side effects of psychiatric drugs are related to unwanted antagonism at cholinergic, adrenergic or histaminic receptors (Table 10.6). The prescription of multiple drugs can result in additive effects.

Anticholinergic side effects are particularly important in older people, especially in those with cognitive impairment. Many elderly people will already be prescribed one or more drugs with a degree of anticholinergic activity (e.g. antiemetic for dizzy spells). Adding another drug with anticholinergic effects (e.g. a tricyclic antidepressant) may put the patient at significant risk of confusion or other anticholinergic effects.

Serotonin or dopamine receptors are often the targets of psychiatric drugs. Their actions at these receptors can have adverse as well as beneficial effects (Table 10.7). These side effects are discussed further in the sections on antidepressant and antipsychotic drugs.

Table 10.7 Serotonergic side effects and effects of dopaminergic antagonism

Serotonergic side effects	Effects of dopaminergic antagonism
Nausea*	Extrapyramidal side effects
Diarrhoea*	– akathisia
Anxiety*	– dystonia
Insomnia*	– Parkinsonism**
Headaches*	– tardive dyskinesia**
Sweating	
Sexual dysfunction	
Serotonin syndrome	Hyperprolactinaemia
	– gynaecomastia
	– galactorrhoea
	Neuroleptic malignant syndrome

*Tend to occur at start of treatment with SSRIs and subside after two weeks of taking treatment
**Elderly may be particularly susceptible

Interactions

Drug interactions can be based on pharmacokinetic or pharmacodynamic mechanisms. Pharmacodynamic interactions relate to the actions of the drugs at specific receptors, for example:

- Additive anticholinergic side effects of amitriptyline and prochlorperazine

- Increased risk of gastrointestinal bleeding when NSAIDs and SSRIs are prescribed together

- Serotonin syndrome when SSRIs are taken with MAOIs, selegiline (see page 175)

- Antagonism of the action of cholinesterase inhibitors (e.g. donepezil) by drugs with anticholinergic side effects (e.g. amitriptyline).

Examples of pharmacokinetic interactions are given in Table 10.8.

Cytochrome P450 enzymes

The cytochrome P450 (CYP450) system comprises over 30 enzymes that are predominantly sited in the liver and play a key role in drug metabolism. The four main subtypes are 2D6, 2C, 1A2 and 3A4. There is some genetic variation between individuals with respect to activity levels within the different groups, and ageing may impair activity.

Many interactions involving drugs used in psychiatry involve the CYP450 system, because many psychotropic drugs are either inhibitors or substrates of one or more of the enzymes (see Appendix 4). Smoking induces the activity of CYP1A2 and so increases the metabolism of its substrates (hence smokers tend to have lower plasma clozapine levels for a given dose).

Table 10.8 Examples of pharmacokinetic interactions with drugs used in psychiatry

Mechanism	Example of drug interaction
Absorption	Drugs with anticholinergic side effects will slow intestinal motility and therefore delay onset of action of hypnotic drugs
Distribution	Displacement of warfarin from plasma protein by certain antibiotics and possibly psychotropic drugs with high protein binding (e.g. fluoxetine)
Metabolism	Inhibition of cytochrome P450 enzymes by many SSRIs
Elimination	Excretion of lithium is reduced by spironolactone, leading to increased plasma lithium levels

Antidepressant drugs

Antidepressants are as effective at treating depression in elderly patients as they are in younger patients. Depression in older people is often under-treated or not treated at all, in part because of concerns about the potential for adverse effects of drugs. Whilst precautions must be taken when prescribing antidepressants in the elderly, there is no reason for depression to remain untreated or inadequately treated on these grounds.

There is no single drug that is the best to use. The evidence points towards SSRIs and tricyclic antidepressants as being the most effective classes in depression, although the safer side effect profile of the SSRIs usually makes them first choice.

The choice of drug is tailored to the needs of the patient, and any co-morbid illness or medications already prescribed are taken into account. In some situations the side effect of a drug is actually desirable, for example a depressed patient with anorexia might benefit from the weight gain caused by mirtazapine.

Onset of action and duration of treatment

There are important differences between older and younger adults in terms of the onset of action of antidepressant drugs and also the duration of maintenance treatment:

- It may take six to eight weeks of treatment before the onset of antidepressant action in the elderly

- Older patients have an equally good response to antidepressants but they experience higher rates of relapse of depression

- Maintenance treatment therefore needs to be longer than for young adults.

An antidepressant therefore needs to be given for at least six weeks before it is decided that it has not been effective. In terms of maintenance, treatment is kept at the same dose and can be withdrawn one to two years after recovery from a single episode, but this is not an absolute. In elderly people, particularly those at high risk of relapse, treatment should be continued for several years, if not for life Management of depression is covered in more detail (page 68).

Selective serotonin reuptake inhibitors (SSRIs)

Mode of action

SSRIs increase serotonergic transmission by blocking the serotonin reuptake pump. Adaptive changes in receptor sensitivity and numbers that occur over several weeks may further increase synaptic 5-HT and account for the delay in therapeutic effect. SSRIs have minimal effects on other receptors, and their relatively safe side-effect profile makes them first line drugs for treatment of depression in the elderly.

Doses

Table 10.9   SSRI doses in the elderly (for depression)

Drug	Starting dose (mg/day)	Maintenance dose (mg/day)	Available as liquid
Citalopram:			
Tablets	10–20	20–40*	✓
Liquid (drops)	8–16	16–32*	
Escitalopram	5*	5–10*	×
Fluoxetine	20	20*	✓
Fluvoxamine	100	100	×
Paroxetine	20	20–40*	✓
Sertraline	50	50–100	×

*Lower than recommended adult doses
Sources: British National Formulary September 2007, Maudsley Prescribing Guidelines 2007

Other licensed uses

Many SSRIs are used in disorders other than depression, including anxiety disorders, obsessive compulsive disorder, post-traumatic stress disorder and bulimia nervosa. The most effective doses may vary in these cases and there may be differences in effectiveness between individual drugs.

Side effects and toxicity

In general the SSRIs all have similar side effects, the most common and important are listed in Table 10.10. SSRIs need to be used with caution where there is a history of bleeding disorder, particularly gastrointestinal bleeding. Paroxetine can cause mild anticholinergic side effects. In comparison with other antidepressants, SSRIs are very safe in overdose. The exception is citalopram where convulsions, ECG abnormalities and deaths have been reported but overall lethality is low.

Interactions

SSRIs must never be used together with monoamine oxidase inhibitors (MAOIs) because of the high risk of serotonin syndrome. A sufficient wash-out period is needed

Table 10.10   Side effects of SSRIs

Side effect	Notes
Nausea	Tend to occur early in treatment and subside within weeks
Diarrhoea	Try reducing dose and titrating up again slowly
Anxiety	Nausea may be reduced if taken with food
Insomnia	
Headaches	
Sweating	
Fine tremor	Relatively common
	True extrapyramidal symptoms can occur but rare
Sexual dysfunction	Can be a difficult subject for patients to raise
	May affect compliance
Reduced seizure threshold	Still relatively safe in epilepsy
	Caution with electroconvulsive therapy (ECT)
	– prolonged seizures reported with fluoxetine
Hypomania or mania	Caution if history of hypomania or mania
	Contraindicated in manic phase
Hyponatraemia	Elderly are particularly susceptible (see text, page 176)
Serotonin syndrome	See text (page 175)
Weight changes	Fluoxetine leads to ⇓ appetite and weight
	Other SSRIs tend to increase appetite and weight

when switching from one to the other (see below). Interactions with SSRIs via the cytochrome P450 enzyme system are common (see Appendix 4). These and other important interactions are summarised in Table 10.11. Citalopram has the least effect on CYP450 enzymes, the lowest level of plasma protein binding and is the least likely of the SSRIs to interact adversely with other drugs.

Stopping

When an SSRI has been taken for more than five to six weeks, a withdrawal syndrome can develop if it is stopped abruptly (Box 10.5). In general the drug should be withdrawn over a period of four weeks or more before stopping, unless a serious adverse event has occurred. Fluoxetine is the exception to this, because of its long half-life (Table 10.12). Withdrawal symptoms are more likely with drugs that have shorter half-lives, for example paroxetine. The half-lives given in Table 10.12 may be prolonged in elderly people, especially in renal or hepatic impairment.

Table 10.11 SSRI interactions with other drugs

SSRI interaction	Notes
MAOIs	High risk of serotonin syndrome Absolutely contraindicated in combination

Drugs metabolised by CYP450 enzymes	See Appendix 4. Fluoxetine and fluvoxamine particularly implicated, may increase levels and risk of toxicity of:
	  – tricyclic antidepressants
	  – antipsychotics
	  – carbamazepine
	  – theophylline
	  – warfarin (monitor INR)
	Citalopram usually safest choice

NSAIDs	Increased risk of gastrointestinal bleeding
Haloperidol	Increased risk of extrapyramidal side effects (May also be ⇑ drug level due to CYP450 inhibition)
Lithium	Increased risk of tremor and other CNS effects, possibly increased risk of toxicity

Antiepileptics	Interactions are complicated
	  – SSRIs antagonise anticonvulsant effect
	  – some SSRIs increase plasma levels of some anticonvulsants via CYP450 interactions

Antiparkinsonian drugs	Use of SSRIs with selegiline (a monoamine oxidase B inhibitor) can lead to serotonin syndrome

INR International normalised ratio   MAOI monoamine oxidase inhibitor CYP450 cytochrome P450
NSAIDs non-steroidal anti-inflammatory drugs

Box 10.5   Features of the SSRI withdrawal syndrome

Nausea and vomiting

Anorexia

Dizziness

Headache

Anxiety

Insomnia

Paraesthesia

"Electric-shock" sensations

Table 10.12   Approximate half lives of the SSRIs based on healthy adults. Half-lives may be prolonged in elderly people but there are no absolute data

SSRI	Half-life
Fluoxetine	4–6 days
Norfluoxetine (metabolite of fluoxetine)	7–15 days
Citalopram	35 hours
Escitalopram	30 hours
Sertraline	26 hours
Paroxetine	21 hours
Fluvoxamine	15 hours

The existence of this withdrawal syndrome does not mean that SSRIs are "addictive," and it is important to explain this to patients who may be concerned about becoming dependent on medication.

Switching

Care needs to be taken when switching antidepressants (Table 10.13), in part because of the risk of serotonin syndrome. When switching from an SSRI to an MAOI, there must be no cross-taper at all and a wash-out period of at least two weeks (five weeks for fluoxetine) is required.

Table 10.13   Switching from SSRIs to other antidepressant drugs

Drug switching to	Comments
Another SSRI	In general can stop first drug and start second next day Fluoxetine: stop for seven days before starting second drug at low dose
MAOI	Withdraw SSRI then stop, start MAOI after 2 weeks Fluoxetine: stop and wait for ≥5 weeks before starting MAOI
TCA	Cross-taper cautiously over a month or so Fluoxetine: stop and wait seven days, start TCA at very low dose
Venlafaxine	Stop SSRI then start venlafaxine at lowest possible dose next day Fluoxetine: stop and wait seven days then as above
Mirtazapine	Cross-taper cautiously over a month or so Fluoxetine: stop for seven days then start mirtazapine cautiously

MAOI monoamine oxidase inhibitor   TCA tricyclic antidepressant   SSRI selective serotonin reuptake inhibitor

Table 10.14 Doses of tricyclic antidepressants in the elderly

Drug	Starting dose (mg/day)	Maintenance dose (mg/day)	Available as liquid
Amitriptyline	25	100–150	√
Clomipramine	10	30–75	×
Dosulepin	50	75–150	×
Imipramine	10	30–50	×
Lofepramine	70	140–210	√
Nortryptiline	30	30–50	×
Trimipramine	75	75–150	×

Sources: British National Formulary September 2007, Maudsley Prescribing Guidelines 2007

Tricyclic antidepressants

Tricyclic antidepressants (TCAs) are effective in the treatment of depression although the range and frequency of side effects mean that they are no longer used as first line drugs. Some TCAs are used in the treatment of anxiety disorders, PTSD and obsessive compulsive disorders (particularly clomipramine) as well as in the management of emotional lability, chronic headache and pain (e.g. amitriptyline).

Mode of action

TCAs act by inhibiting the reuptake of serotonin and/or noradrenaline via effects on transporter proteins. Adaptive changes in the numbers and sensitivity of noradrenergic and serotonergic receptors that further increase synaptic levels of these neurotransmitters probably account for the delay in antidepressant effect. The blockade of acetylcholine, histamine, and α_1-adrenergic receptors does not contribute to the antidepressant effect and is responsible for the majority of side effects caused by TCAs.

The individual TCAs each have different levels of affinity for the different reuptake sites. Most affect both serotonin and noradrenanaline reuptake, although lofepramine is a relatively selective noradrenaline reuptake inhibitor and clomipramine is relatively selective for serotonin reuptake. This is believed to be the reason behind its effectiveness in the management of anxiety disorders and OCD.

Dose

The inter-individual variability in pharmacokinetics of TCAs is markedly increased in old age, with up to a 49-fold variation in TCA levels between different individuals.

Table 10.15 Summary of common and/or important side effects of tricyclic antidepressants

Action	Effect
Anticholinergic effects	Dry mouth
	Blurred vision
	Constipation
	Urinary retention
	Confusion
	Drowsiness
Antihistaminic effects	Sedation
	Weight gain
Anti-α_1 adrenergic effects	Hypotension
	Dizziness
	Sexual dysfunction
Other actions	Cardiac arrhythmias
	Heart block
	Seizures
	Rashes

TCAs should be started at lower doses in the elderly and titrated up cautiously according to clinical effects.

Side effects and toxicity

All TCAs cause varying degrees of anticholinergic, anti α_1-adrenergic and antihistaminic side effects (Table 10.15) and should be used with caution in the elderly. The membrane-stabilising properties of this group of drugs can also lead to cardiac arrhythmias. Amitriptyline is particularly known for its anticholinergic effects and dosulepin for its cardiotoxic effects. Lofepramine has relatively mild side effects and low cardiotoxicity and so is one of the safest of the TCAs. However, postural hypotension can be a problem.

Sedation may be seen as an advantage in patients with insomnia or agitation but must be balanced against the risk of confusion and falls. Amitriptyline and clomipramine are the most sedative of the TCAs whereas lofepramine, imipramine and nortriptyline are far less so. The use of TCAs in the management of insomnia in the absence of any other indication is not justified.

TCAs are toxic in overdose; severe cardiac arrhythmias and even asystole can occur. Suicidality must be considered when prescribing, other cautions and contraindications are listed in Table 10.16.

Table 10.16 Some important cautions and contraindications for tricyclic antidepressants

Contraindications	Cautions
Post myocardial infarction	Closed angle glaucoma
Cardiac arrhythmias	Urinary retention (NB prostatism)
Heart block	Epilepsy/ECT
Mania	Thyroid disease
	History of mania
	Hepatic impairment

Table 10.17 Drug interactions with TCAs

Drug	Notes
MAOIs and serotonergic drugs	Risk of serotonin syndrome, most relevant with clomipramine
Drugs with anticholinergic activity	Additive anticholinergic effects
Inhibitors/inducers of CYP450 enzymes	For example, SSRIs increase plasma levels of TCAs
Antiarrhythmics	Increased risk of arrhythmias
Alcohol	Increased sedative effect

Interactions

Many potential drug interactions with TCAs involve the cytochrome P450 system (Appendix 4). Some of the most important interactions are highlighted in Table 10.17.

Stopping and switching

As with the SSRIs, TCAs should be withdrawn slowly rather than stopped abruptly. Varying degrees of caution are needed when switching to another antidepressant (Table 10.18).

Monoamine oxidase inhibitors

Monoamine oxidase inhibitors (MAOIs) are used in the management of depression, anxiety states and OCD when other drugs have been ineffective. They may be more effective than other drugs in the management of atypical depression.

Side effects, drug interactions and a potentially life-threatening hypertensive crisis if tyramine-rich foods are ingested mean that caution is needed when these drugs are used in any patients, particularly the elderly.

Table 10.18   Switching from tricyclic to other antidepressants

Drug switching to	Comments
Another TCA **Venlafaxine** **Mirtazapine**	Cross-taper cautiously
MAOI	Withdraw then wait one week before starting MAOI
SSRIs **Trazodone** **Reboxetine**	Half the dose of the TCA and add in the new drug, then withdraw the TCA slowly

Source: Maudsley Prescribing Guidelines 2007

Mode of action

MAOIs act via inhibition of monoamine oxidase (MAO). There are two important MAO enzymes, MAO-A is preferentially involved in the metabolism of serotonin and noradrenaline, and MAO-B in dopamine metabolism. Inhibition of MAO is believed to increase both the storage and release of these monoamine neurotransmitters, hence increasing neurotransmission. Monoamine oxidase enzymes are also found outside of the CNS, for example in the gut wall and liver, and inhibition of these enzymes is responsible for the "cheese reaction" (see below).

Table 10.19   Actions of the monoamine oxidase inhibitors

Drug	Action
Moclobemide	Reversible inhibition of MAO-A
Phenelzine **Tranylcypromine** **Isocarboxazid**	Irreversible inhibition of MAO-A and MAO-B
Selegiline	Reversible inhibition of MAO-B

MAO monoamine oxidase

Phenelzine, tranylcypromine and isocarboxazid are all irreversible inhibitors of both MAO-A and MAO-B. Tranylcypromine has stimulant properties and is chemically re-lated to amphetamine. Moclobemide is often classified separately from MAOIs as a reversible inhibitor of monoamine oxidase A (RIMA). Selegiline is used in Parkinson's disease and not in depression.

Doses

Table 10.20 Starting and maintenance doses of MAOIs in mg/day

Drug	Starting dose (mg/day)	Maintenance dose (mg/day)	Available as liquid
Phenelzine	15	15–45	×
Tranylcypromine	10	10–30	×
Isocarboxazid	30 (for six weeks)	5–10	×
Moclobemide	150	150–600	×

Side effects

MAOIs are used in the elderly only with great caution. The exception is moclobemide, which is relatively safe and well tolerated. Table 10.21 gives a summary of the main side effects and contraindications.

Table 10.21 Important side effects and contraindications for MAOIs

Drug (s)	Side effects	Contraindications
Phenelzine and isocarboxazid	Sedation Postural hypotension Hepatotoxicity Sweating Dry mouth Blurred vision Constipation Agitation/tremor Psychosis	Hepatic impairment Cerebrovascular disease Congestive cardiac failure Phaeochromocytoma
Tranylcypromine	As above but: Insomnia (not sedation) Less hepatotoxic	As above
Moclobemide	Insomnia Dizziness Gastrointestinal upset Headache Restlessness and agitation	Acute confusional states Phaeochromocytoma

Table 10.22 Important food and drug interactions with MAOIs

Food interactions	Drug interactions
Cheese (especially mature) Yeast and protein extract (marmite etc.) Chianti wine	Sympathomimetic amines (often in over-the-counter cough and cold medicines)
Fava or broad bean pods Hung game Chicken liver	SSRIs and other serotonergic antidepressants (serotonin syndrome)
Pickled herring Smoked fish	Opiates Insulin (increased sensitivity)

Interactions

Food   Inhibition of gut MAO can lead to a potentially fatal hypertensive crisis if foods containing tyramine are ingested. Tyramine is normally broken down by intestinal MAO, and if this is blocked then high levels are able to enter the circulation and exert hypertensive effects. Foods to avoid are shown in Table 10.22.

Drugs   A number of drugs must be avoided in patients taking a MAOI, and these include any that are metabolised by monoamine oxidase enzymes (Table 10.22).

Stopping and switching

MAOIs should be withdrawn gradually before stopping. When switching to another antidepressant, moclobemide can be withdrawn and the new drug started 24 hours later. For phenelzine, isocarboxazid and tranylcypromine a gap of two weeks is needed.

When switching to an MAOI from any other antidepressant that affects serotonin reuptake, the original drug must be given adequate time to leave the body. Further details are given in the relevant antidepressant sections.

Trazodone

Trazodone is classified as a serotonin antagonist and reuptake inhibitor (SARI). The 2006 Cochrane review of antidepressants in the elderly found it comparable to the SSRIs in both effectiveness and side-effect profile. It acts by inhibiting serotonin reuptake and also has effects at specific 5-HT receptors.

Dose

In the elderly the starting dose is 100 mg (in divided doses or single dose at night) and the maintenance dose is usually 150 mg.

Side effects

Trazodone has potent effects at histamine receptors and some effect at α_1-adrenergic receptors. There are no anticholinergic effects. Side effects include considerable sedation, postural hypotension, priapism and cardiotoxicity. Trazodone is relatively safe in overdose.

Interactions

The effects of any sedative drug will be exacerbated by trazodone. Serotonin syndrome is possible with MAOIs although unlikely.

Stopping and switching

Table 10.23 Switching from trazodone to other antidepressant drugs

Drug switching to	Comments
SSRIs **Reboxetine**★ **Venlafaxine**★★	Withdraw then start new drug
TCAs **Mirtazapine**	Cross taper cautiously
MAOIs	Withdraw then wait at least one week

★Start at 2 mg/day   ★★Start at 37.5 mg/day

Venlafaxine

Venlafaxine is a serotonin and noradrenaline reuptake inhibitor (SNRI) and has relatively few effects on other receptors. In lower doses it is mainly a serotonin reuptake inhibitor. The starting dose in the elderly is usually 37.5 mg daily and the normal maintenance dose is 75–150 mg daily. A modified release preparation is available which may help adherence.

Side effects

The most common and important side effects of venlafaxine are given in Box 10.6. It is important to note that venlafaxine can cause or exacerbate hypertension, particularly at higher doses. It should be avoided in hypertension and heart disease. Blood pressure must be monitored regularly during treatment.

Box 10.6 Side effects of venlafaxine	
Drowsiness	Nausea
Dizziness	Sexual dysfunction
Headache	Sweating
Dry mouth	Anorexia
Insomnia	Hypertension
Nervousness	Aesthenia
Constipation	Seizures

Venlafaxine is relatively safe in overdose and fatalities are rare.

Interactions

Co-administration of venlafaxine with MAOIs carries a high risk of serotonin syndrome and is avoided. Venlafaxine is metabolised by the cytochrome P450 system (Appendix 4).

Stopping and switching

As with SSRIs, abrupt cessation of venlafaxine leads to discontinuation symptoms. The half-life is relatively short and the dosage should be gradually reduced before stopping. When switching to MAOIs, venlafaxine should be withdrawn and the new drug started after a week or more. For all other antidepressants cautious cross-tapering with low doses of the new drug is generally safe.

Mirtazapine

Mirtazapine is classified as a noradrenergic and specific serotonergic antidepressant. It blocks noradrenergic α_2-autoreceptors resulting in increased noradrenaline and serotonin release from nerve terminals. It is a popular drug for treating depression in the elderly in cases where sedation and weight gain are desirable.

Dose

The starting dose is 15 mg daily, and the normal maintenance dose is 15–45 mg.

Table 10.24 Side effects of mirtazapine

Common	Less common	Rare
Sedation	Dizziness	Postural hypotension
Weight gain	Headache	Tremor
Oedema		Muscle and joint pains
		Agranulocytosis

Side effects

Mirtazapine does not have significant anticholinergic side effects and does not tend to cause postural hypotension. Side effects are summarised in Table 10.24. Mirtazapine is safe in overdose, causing sedation and very occasionally seizures but no cardiac effects. Patients must be warned to report fever, sore throat or any other signs of infection during treatment because of the (rare) possibility of agranulocytosis. If this is suspected, stop the drug and perform a full blood count immediately.

Interactions

Mirtazapine has relatively few interactions; the most important is with the MAOIs. There may be additive effects with other drugs that cause sedation.

Stopping and switching

As with most antidepressants, mirtazapine should be withdrawn gradually before stopping. When switching, mirtazapine is stopped and then the new antidepressant can usually be started straight away. The exception is the MAOIs, where at least a week is needed in between.

Reboxetine

Reboxetine is a noradrenergic reuptake inhibitor. There is little information available regarding its use in the elderly and at present it is not recommended. In younger adults its effectiveness and tolerability is probably comparable to the SSRIs.

St John's Wort

St John's Wort (extract of Hypericum perforatum) is seen by many as a "natural" remedy for depression. It is available to buy over the counter in UK pharmacies. St John's Wort appears to have monoamine oxidase A and B inhibitory properties and probably inhibits the reuptake of noradrenaline, serotonin and dopamine. It may be an inducer of cytochrome P450 enzymes and other drug interactions may occur because of the MAOI activity. Interactions with anticoagulants are particularly important.

It is quite possible that St John's Wort is an effective and safe treatment for mild to moderate depression, but it is not recommended by NICE because there is inadequate evidence regarding its efficacy and safety and the exact nature of the active ingredient is not understood.

Patients taking St John's Wort who wish to start an antidepressant drug must first withdraw the St John's Wort. The two should not be taken simultaneously because of the risk of serotonin syndrome or other interactions.

Serotonin syndrome

The serotonin syndrome is a rare, life-threatening syndrome (Box 10.7) that is caused by serotonergic drugs. It usually occurs in the context of interactions between antidepressants, and combining any serotonergic drug with an MAOI is extremely dangerous. Diagnosis is clinical and supported by high plasma creatinine kinase (CK) levels. Management is supportive; medical colleagues should be involved early if there is any suspicion of serotonin syndrome.

Box 10.7   Features of the serotonin syndrome

Restlessness

Fever

Sweating

Diarrhoea

Tremor

Shivering

Myoclonus

Hyperreflexia

Confusion

Convulsions

From: Sternbach H (1991) The serotonin syndrome *AJP* 148: 705–713

Hyponatraemia

Hyponatraemia is common in elderly people (Box 10.8) and it can be induced or exacerbated by any antidepressant drug, particularly the SSRIs. It possibly occurs as a result of inappropriate antidiuretic hormone release. Patients who develop hyponatraemia usually do so within the first few weeks of starting the drug.

Older people on antidepressants should be monitored clinically for signs of hyponatraemia (Box 10.9) and there is an argument for regular serum electrolyte monitoring. A serum sodium level of above 125 mmol/L can be managed by withdrawing the drug and monitoring levels; serum sodium below 125 mmol/L warrants referral to a medical team. An alternative antidepressant can be prescribed, preferably one with a less potent serotonergic action.

Box 10.8   Risk factors for hyponatraemia

Old age

Female sex

Low body weight

Renal impairment

Physical illness

Medication (e.g. loop diuretics, carbamazepine)

Box 10.9   Clinical features of hyponatraemia

Confusion

Nausea

Cramps

Muscle weakness

Oedema

Seizures

Antidepressants and co-morbid illness

Many older people with depression will also suffer from a physical illness. Some antidepressants are particularly dangerous in certain conditions where others have been shown to be both safe and effective. Table 10.25 summarises drugs to avoid and suggestions for safer options, based on the available evidence.

Table 10.25   Antidepressant drug use in co-morbid illness

Co-morbid condition	Safer options	Avoid
Hypertension **Gastritis/peptic ulcer**	SSRI	Venlafaxine SSRIs
Post myocardial infarction **Arrhythmias**	Sertraline SSRI Moclobemide	TCAs TCAs
Heart failure	Citalopram	TCAs Trazodone Venlafaxine
Dementia	Citalopram Fluoxetine (if adherence concerns, long half-life)	TCAs
Stroke	Citalopram Nortriptyline	MAOIs
Narrow angle glaucoma	SSRIs (but reports of worsening of glaucoma with paroxetine, fluoxetine)	TCAs
Urinary retention/ **prostatic disease**	SSRIs	TCAs
Renal impairment★	Citalopram Sertraline	Lofepramine
Hepatic impairment★	Citalopram Paroxetine Imipramine	TCAs MAOIs Sertraline
Epilepsy	SSRIs Trazodone Moclobemide	TCAs
Parkinson's disease	SSRIs★★	MAOIs**

*Refer to prescribing guidelines whenever prescribing in renal or hepatic impairment; dose reductions are often necessary
**See text

Cardiovascular disease

TCAs are best avoided in cardiovascular disease. SSRIs are usually the safest option for patients with arrhythmias. Sertraline has been shown to be both safe and effective in the period following myocardial infarction. Hypertension is often exacerbated by venlafaxine and so is avoided in hypertensive patients. Drugs that cause postural hypotension are dangerous in heart failure and so TCAs, trazodone and venlafaxine are best avoided.

Stroke

For depressed patients who have recently had a stroke, SSRIs and nortriptyline have been shown to be safe and effective. Citalopram is the least likely to interact with warfarin.

Parkinson's disease

Both Parkinson's disease and the drugs used in its management pose a challenge when deciding on an antidepressant. SSRIs are generally safe and effective but combination with selegiline (a MAOI) is unsafe. TCAs are also effective but tend not to be well tolerated. The anticholinergic effects of TCAs may worsen cognitive function and $\alpha 1$-adrenoreceptor blockade can exacerbate the autonomic dysfunction experienced by many patients with Parkinson's disease. MAOIs interact with selegiline and can cause a hypertensive crisis with levodopa.

Epilepsy

Most antidepressants cause a dose-related reduction in seizure threshold and those with sedative properties tend to have a more significant effect. Moclobemide, trazodone and SSRIs are good choices in epilepsy and have little proconvulsive effect. Interactions with antiepileptic drugs via the cytochrome P450 system can be a problem with SSRIs. TCAs should be avoided altogether.

Dementia

Depression in dementia is discussed on page 72.

Summary of antidepressant side effects

Table 10.26 Summary of side effects of antidepressants

Drug class	Drug	Anti-cholinergic effects	Sedation	Hypotension	Weight gain
SSRI	Fluoxetine	+/−	−	−	−*
	Citalopram	+/−	+/−	−	+/−
	Escitalopram	+/−	+/−	−	+/−
	Sertraline	+/−	−	−	−
	Paroxetine	+	+	−	+
	Fluvoxamine	+/−	+	−	−
TCA	Amitriptyline	+++	+++	+++	++
	Clomipramine	++	++	+++	
	Dothiepin	++	+++	+++	
	Imipramine	+++	++	+++	++
	Lofepramine	+	+	+	++
	Nortriptyline	+	+	++	++
	Trimipramine	++	+++	+++	++
SNRI	Venlafaxine	+/−	+/−	−	−
NASSA	Mirtazapine	+/−	+++	−	++
RIMA	Moclobemide	+/−	−	−	−
MAOI	Phenelzene	+/−	+	+	++
	Tranylcypromine		−**	+	+
	Isocarboxazid		+	++	++
SARI	Trazodone	−	+++	++	−

− minimal or absent   + mild   ++ moderate   +++ severe or extremely common
*Fluoxetine often causes weight loss
**Tranylcypromine can cause both sedation and activation

Lithium

Indications

Uses of lithium include:

- Treatment and prophylaxis of mania

- Prophylaxis in bipolar affective disorder

- Prophylaxis in recurrent depressive disorder

- Lithium augmentation in treatment-resistant depression.

Mode of action

Lithium is the smallest alkaline cation. It can substitute for sodium, potassium, magnesium and calcium. Its effects are believed to relate to actions involving second messenger systems and 5-HT receptor regulation.

Pharmacokinetics

After ingestion, there is an initial peak in plasma lithium levels followed by a slower phase. The processes behind this can be summarised as:

1. Rapid intestinal absorption with plasma level peak at 1–4 hours.
2. Lithium leaves plasma via renal elimination or distribution throughout body fluids and cells.
3. Slow release from cells ⇒ lower plasma level than initial peak.

The elimination half-life in young healthy adults is 7–20 hours, increasing in the elderly to around 30 hours. Any reduction of renal blood flow or impairment of renal function will increase plasma lithium levels during regular administration.

Within the kidney lithium is excreted and then partially reabsorbed in competition with sodium. Reabsorption and hence plasma levels are increased by:

- Dehydration: more water and therefore lithium is reabsorbed.

- Salt depletion: less sodium filtered ⇒ more lithium is reabsorbed (e.g. diet, sweating, fever).

- Thiazide and loop diuretics (affect sodium loss).

Box 10.10   Factors that increase plasma lithium concentration

Renal impairment

Hypotension

Heart failure

Dehydration

Sodium depletion

Thiazide and loop diuretics

Table 10.27 Monitoring requirements during lithium therapy in elderly patients

Timing	Comments
Before starting treatment	U&E TFT ECG
First plasma level	Five to seven days after starting treatment (steady state reached)
Weekly	Lithium levels until stable therapeutic level reached
Three monthly (at least)	Lithium levels U&E Initial period of treatment
Six monthly	TFT U&E Lithium levels (Once patient well stabilised)
Yearly	Calcium if long-term treatment
Additional monitoring of plasma levels	Intercurrent illness Potential drug interactions

U&E urea and electrolytes   TFT thyroid function tests

Monitoring

Lithium has a narrow therapeutic window and there is considerable variation in plasma levels between individuals. Regular monitoring is mandatory (Table 10.27). Levels are taken 12 hours or more after the dose, after the initial peak.

Dose

The dose requirement in the elderly is usually one third to one half of that required in younger adults. It is best to start with 200 mg daily and gradually increase until a stable therapeutic level is reached. In young adults this is 0.4–1 mmol/l. In elderly patients it is best to aim for the lower end of the range (0.4–0.6 mmol/l). It is unusual to need more than 600 mg per day in older people.

Side effects

The elderly are more susceptible to the side effects of lithium than younger patients. A summary is given in Box 10.11, with more details below.

Box 10.11   Side effects of lithium

Nausea

Diarrhoea

Hypothyroidism

Thirst and polydipsia

Metallic taste

Fine tremor

Renal impairment

Arrhythmias

Exacerbation of skin conditions

Weight gain

Leucocytosis (benign and reversible)

Parkinsonian symptoms (unusual, elderly more vulnerable)

Early side effects

Some degree of abdominal discomfort, nausea, diarrhoea and fine tremor are quite common early in treatment and often disappear. Dividing the doses may help in these cases. More severe diarrhoea and/or vomiting suggest toxicity.

Thyroid changes

Laboratory markers of hypothyroidism are raised in up to 25 % of elderly patients taking lithium and clinical hypothyroidism occurs in 5–10 %. This can be easily treated with thyroxine. Thyroid function will usually return to normal levels within a few months of stopping lithium but this may have significant consequences for the patient.

Cardiac side effects

T-wave flattening and arrhythmias can occur and an ECG is necessary before starting lithium treatment. Cardiac disease is not an absolute contraindication for treatment with lithium but it is a good idea to discuss the issue with a cardiologist.

Renal impairment

Lithium can cause direct damage to the kidney but this generally occurs with toxicity and is unusual with careful monitoring of plasma levels. Lithium can be used with caution in mild renal impairment but is avoided in moderate or severe cases.

Table 10.28   Features of lithium toxicity

Mild	Moderate	Severe
Anorexia	Vomiting	Incontinence
Nausea	Ataxia	Muscle weakness/twitching
Diarrhoea	Coarse tremor	Spasticity
Worsening fine tremor	Dysarthria	Arrhythmias
	Drowsiness	Seizures
	Disorientation	Coma

Toxicity

Older people are more at risk of toxicity because of the higher likelihood of renal impairment, polypharmacy and co-morbidity. Poor adherence may result in a low plasma level recording; the doctor may then increase the dose in error, leading to toxicity.

If toxicity is suspected, urgently check plasma lithium and U&E levels and involve medical colleagues early. Mild cases may be managed by stopping lithium and increasing oral fluids but more severe toxicity may require diuresis or haemodialysis.

Interactions

The most important interactions with lithium are those that increase its plasma level or toxicity (Table 10.29). Lithium also increases the risk of extrapyramidal side effects with antipsychotic drugs.

Anticonvulsant mood stabilisers

Valproate and carbamazepine are widely used as mood stabilisers in both younger adults and the elderly. There are few studies of their efficacy compared to either placebo or lithium in elderly bipolar patients. Valproate is probably more effective than carbamazepine in acute mania and may have a safer side-effect profile.

Table 10.29 Drugs that increase plasma level or toxicity of lithium

Drugs that increase plasma lithium levels	Drugs that increase lithium toxicity
Diuretics (thiazide > loop)	Haloperidol
ACE inhibitors	Chlorpromazine
NSAIDs	Clozapine
	Carbamazepine
	Phenytoin
	Metronidazole
	Some antiarrhythmics

Valproate

Valproate increases GABA neurotransmission although exactly how it achieves its mood stabilising effect is unclear. It is available as sodium valproate and semisodium valproate. Valproate is metabolised by the liver and has a half-life of 8–20 hours. A slow-release form of sodium valproate (Epilim Chrono) allows once-daily dosing. Liver function must be tested before starting treatment.

Dose

The initial dose of sodium valproate is 200 mg b.d. (or semisodium valproate 250 mg b.d., or Epilim Chrono 500 mg o.d.), increased as necessary. This can be guided by plasma levels (12 hours after dose); the therapeutic range is 50–100 mg/l. In bipolar affective disorder the usual dose is 1000 mg per day.

Side effects

Valproate is usually well tolerated by older people. Most of the common side effects (Table 10.30) are transient. The slow release form may be associated with fewer of these effects. One disadvantage of using valproate over lithium in bipolar affective disorder is the higher risk of weight gain.

A transient increase in liver enzymes often occurs in patients taking valproate. In most cases liver function tests (LFTs) and prothrombin time can be monitored until the results return to normal but treatment should be stopped if clinically significant side effects develop or prothrombin time is increased.

Interactions

Valproate has complex interactions with other anticonvulsants and may also increase levels of TCAs and MAOIs. It potentiates the activity of aspirin and

Table 10.30   Side effects of valproate

Common	Rare
Nausea	Ataxia
Vomiting	Confusion
Mild sedation	Headache
Weight gain	Pancytopaenia
Hair loss	Platelet dysfunction
	Pancreatitis
	Hepatic dysfunction

warfarin; additional INR monitoring is necessary in warfarinised patients starting on valproate.

Carbamazepine

Carbamazepine is a GABA agonist and reduces calcium channel activation, but the mechanism behind its mood stabilising properties is unclear.

Dose

In bipolar affective disorder in the elderly, the dose is initially 50–100 mg b.d., increased slowly up to 600 mg daily.

Side effects

Table 10.31   Side effects of carbamazepine

Common	Unusual
Drowsiness	Agranulocytosis (1 in 20 000)
Agitation*	Aplastic anaemia (1 in 20 000)
Headache	Stevens-Johnson syndrome
Ataxia	
Diplopia	
Nausea	
Transient leucopenia	
Rash (may need to discontinue drug)	
Hyponatraemia (SIADH)	

*Usually only occurs in elderly

Table 10.32 Cytochrome P450 interactions involving carbamazepine

Drugs that increase plasma level of carbamazepine	Drugs that decrease plasma level of carbamazepine	Drugs whose plasma levels are decreased by carbamazepine
SSRIs	Barbiturates	TCAs
Valproate	Phenytoin	Valproate
Verapamil		Warfarin
Erythromycin		
Cimetidine		
Co-proxamol		

The elderly are at increased risk of the above side effects of carbamazepine, particularly neurotoxic effects, agitation and hyponatraemia.

Up to 15 % of patients develop an itchy maculopapular rash within the first few weeks of treatment. In these cases a full blood count must be taken urgently and carbamazepine stopped. Rarely, carbamazepine can cause agranulocytosis and so patients must be warned to report a sore throat or any other sign of infection. The full blood count should be monitored fortnightly during the first two months, and then six-monthly. Sodium levels should also be monitored.

Interactions

Carbamazepine both induces liver enzymes and is metabolised by them, so it increases metabolism of many drugs including itself. Plasma levels of carbamazepine therefore fall after several weeks of treatment. Important interactions are given in Table 10.32. Carbamazepine can also increase the toxicity of lithium.

Antipsychotic drugs

The use of antipsychotic drugs in old age psychiatry is kept to a minimum although there are situations where their use is appropriate. Important considerations when prescribing antipsychotics for elderly people include:

- Lower doses necessary for clinical effect

- Wider variation between individuals in blood levels for a given dose

- Marked increased risk of side effects, low doses necessary

- Risk of drug interactions and co-morbid illness (especially cardiac).

Uses of antipsychotic drugs in the elderly are varied and in some cases there is a limited evidence base. Possible indications include:

- Treatment of psychotic disorders (page 116)

- Treatment of manic illness (page 87)

- Aggression and agitation in delirium (page 251)

- Behavioural and psychiatric symptoms of dementia (page 29)

- Occasionally severe anxiety or OCD (page 107).

Antipsychotic drugs can cause severe extrapyramidal side effects and increase mortality in patients who have dementia with Lewy bodies. The use of olanzapine and risperidone in dementia is associated with an increased risk of stroke, an effect that probably applies to all antipsychotic drugs.

Mechanism of action

Antipsychotic drugs block dopamine receptors and in general the strength of this effect *in vitro* correlates with clinical effectiveness. The D_2 receptor appears to be the most significant in terms of antipsychotic effect although other receptor actions may be important with the atypical antipsychotics, including $5\text{-}HT_2$ antagonism.

Typical and atypical antipsychotic drugs (Table 10.33) differ in that atypical antipsychotics are much less likely to cause extrapyramidal side effects (EPSE, Table 10.34). They may also have more effect on the negative symptoms of schizophrenia.

Dose

Doses vary according to the indication but it is more important than with any other class of drugs that the lowest possible dose is prescribed when starting antipsychotic drugs. Starting doses of 0.5 mg of haloperidol or risperidone may seem low dose compared to those used in general adult psychiatry but are often enough to be effective. It is safer to start low and increase, than to risk potentially serious side effects and reduced adherence.

Side effects

There are many side effects that occur to varying degrees of severity with most antipsychotic drugs. Box 10.12 lists common side effects and Table 10.33 summarises the severity of the main side effects with the different drugs.

Table 10.33 Side effects of antipsychotic drugs

Drug group	Drug name	EPSE	Anti-cholinergic	Increased prolactin	Hypotension	Sedation	Weight gain	Increased QTc
Typicals								
Phenothiazines	Chlorpromazine	+	++	+++	+++	+++	++	++
	Thioridazine	+	+++	++	+++	++	++	+++
	Fluphenazine	+++	+	+++	+	+	+	+
	Trifluoperazine	+++	+	+++	+	++	–	?
Burtyrophenone	Haloperidol	+++	+	+++	+	+	+	+
Thioxanthines	Flupenthixol	++	++	+++	+	+	++	++
	Zuclopenthixol	+++	++	+++	+	++	++	?
Atypicals								
Substituted benzamides	Amisulpiride	+	–	++	–	++	+	–
	Sulpiride	+	–	++	–	++	+	+
Quinolone	Aripriprazole	–/+	–	–	–	–	–	–
Dibenzobenzodiazepine	Clozapine	–/+	+++	–	+++	+++	+++	+
Thienobenzodiazepine	Olanzapine	–/+	+	–/+	+	++	+++	+
Dibenzothiazepine	Quetiapine	–/+	–/+	–/+	+	++	++	++
Benzisoxazole	Risperidone	+	–/+	++	++	+	++	+

– Absent/minimal + low ++ moderate +++ severe or high frequency ? unknown EPSE extrapyramidal side effects
QTc corrected QT interval

Table 10.34 Extrapyramidal side effects (EPSE) and management strategies

EPSE	Description	Time taken to develop	Management
Acute akathisia	Subjective state of inner restlessness. Compulsive motor restlessness, especially of legs	Hours to weeks	Reduce dose Change to atypical Clonazepam* Propanolol*
Parkinsonism	Tremor Rigidity Bradykinesia (e.g., movements, facial expression, flat voice) Salivation	Days to weeks	Reduce dose Change to atypical
Acute dystonia	Muscle spasm, e.g. oculogyric crisis, torticollis	Hours	Anticholinergic drugs orally, i.m. or i.v.
Tardive dyskinesia	Involuntary repetitive, purposeless choreiform orolingual and masticatory movements, e.g. grimacing, tongue protrusion, lip smacking	Months to years 50 % are reversible	Reduce dose or stop Change to atypical Clozapine Tetrabenazine

*Not recommended in elderly

Box 10.12   Side effects of antipsychotic drugs

Extrapyramidal side effects

Anticholinergic effects

Postural hypotension

Hyperprolactinaemia

Sedation

Weight gain

Sexual dysfunction

Impaired glucose tolerance/diabetes

Cardiac effects including QT interval prolongation

Reduction in seizure threshold

Extrapyramidal side effects

Extrapyramidal side effects (EPSE, Table 10.34) may be caused by any antipsychotic drug but are most common with typical antipsychotics. They result from dopaminergic antagonism in the nigrostriatal pathway. The elderly are extremely sensitive to EPSE, especially Parkinsonian symptoms and tardive dyskinesia. In dementia with Lewy bodies these reactions can be particularly severe.

If EPSE occur, the most appropriate action is usually to reduce the dose, stop the antipsychotic, or switch to an atypical drug that is less likely to cause EPSE. Quetiapine, olanzapine or aripiprazole are options in this situation.

Anticholinergic drugs in the treatment of EPSE   Dopamine in the basal ganglia usually acts to inhibit cholinergic neurones. Antipsychotic drugs block the action of dopamine and therefore increase acetylcholine release.

Anticholinergic drugs (procyclidine, benztropine and orphenadrine) can be used in the treatment of certain EPSE (Table 10.33). It is generally better to reduce the antipsychotic dose or change drugs than to use anticholinergic drugs. Side effects of anticholinergic drugs include confusion, visual hallucinations, constipation and urinary retention. Use is avoided in the elderly.

Other management options in EPSE   Benzodiazepines can be used in tardive dyskinesia and akathisia but in the elderly the risk of sedation, confusion and falls often outweighs any potential benefit. Propanolol may also help in akathisia but carries a risk of hypotension and exacerbation of heart failure or lung disease.

Clozapine is the drug most likely to benefit people with tardive dyskinesia but is associated with significant side effects of its own (see below). Tetrabenazine is the only drug licensed in the UK for the treatment of tardive dyskinesia.

Cardiac effects

Many antipsychotic drugs cause an increase in the QT interval (Table 10.33), increasing the risk of arrythmias and sudden cardiac death. Patients particularly at risk are those with pre-existing cardiac disease and those who are administered intramuscular antipsychotics under restraint.

In elderly people it is sensible to take an ECG both before starting treatment and at regular intervals during treatment.

Weight gain and diabetes

Weight gain is a side effect of almost all antipsychotic drugs but is particularly a problem with olanzapine, clozapine and to a lesser extent other atypical antipsychotics. Fasting

Table 10.35   Antipsychotic use in epilepsy

Safer options	Use with caution	Avoid
Sulpiride	Risperidone	Chlorpromazine
Haloperidol	Olanzapine	Clozapine
	Quetiapine	Depot antipsychotics
	Amisulpiride	

plasma glucose and lipids should be checked one to three months after starting treatment and then regularly (at least annually) for the duration of treatment.

Development of glucose intolerance or diabetes contributes to the increased levels of morbidity and mortality already experienced by older psychiatric patients. Recognition and treatment must be proactive.

Seizures

Many antipsychotic drugs lower the seizure threshold; clozapine and chlorpromazine have the strongest effect. In patients who already have epilepsy, sulpiride is probably the safest choice (Table 10.35).

Neuroleptic malignant syndrome

Neuroleptic malignant syndrome (NMS) is a rare but potentially fatal side effect that can occur with any antipsychotic drug. Features include muscle rigidity, pyrexia, sweating, autonomic instability and confusion (Table 10.36).

Management includes stopping the antipsychotic drug, rehydration and supportive therapy. Early liaison with medical colleagues is essential. Dopamine agonists (bromocryptine, dantroline) are sometimes used.

Table 10.36   Features of neuroleptic malignant syndrome

Risk factors	Clinical features	Laboratory findings
High potency drug	Muscle rigidity	Raised creatinine kinase
New drug/dose increase	Fever	Leucocytosis
Agitation	Sweating	Deranged LFTs
Dehydration	Confusion	
Organic brain disease	↓ level of consciousness	
Alcoholism	Fluctuating heart rate	
Hyperthyroidism	Fluctuating BP	

Table 10.37 Advantages and side effects of note of clozapine in the elderly

Advantages	Notable side effects
Effective in many treatment-resistant cases	Sedation
Reduced EPSE	Weight gain
More effective for negative symptoms	Hypotension and falls
Reduced suicide risk	Hypersalivation
May reduce depression/anxiety	Reduced seizure threshold
Effective in psychosis in Parkinson's disease	Agranulocytosis, need for monitoring

Clozapine

Clozapine is effective in the management of treatment-resistant schizophrenia. It is effective but poorly tolerated in the elderly, and has significant side effects that limit its use (Table 10.37). In Parkinson's disease, clozapine has been shown to improve psychosis without worsening Parkinsonism.

All side effects of clozapine increase with age, including agranulocytosis. Patients must be registered with the clozapine monitoring service and require weekly full blood counts for 16 weeks, after which frequency decreases.

Interactions

Table 10.38 Common interactions involving antipsychotic drugs

Drug	Antipsychotic	Comments
TCA	Typical antipsychotics	⇑ plasma level of TCA
Fluoxetine	Haloperidol	⇑ EPSE
SSRI	Clozapine	⇑ plasma level of clozapine
	Risperidone	⇑ plasma level of risperidone
	Quetiapine	⇑ plasma level of quetiapine
Risperidone	Clozapine	⇑ plasma level of clozapine
Lithium	Clozapine or phenothiazines	⇑ lithium toxicity
Cimetidine	Most antipsychotics	⇓ plasma levels of antipsychotics
Anticholinergics	Most antipsychotics	Additive anticholinergic effects
Drugs with sedative effects	Most antipsychotics	Additive sedative effects

TCA tricyclic antidepressant   EPSE extrapyramidal side effects   SSRI selective serotonin reuptake inhibitor

Depot medication

Long-lasting intramuscular injections of antipsychotic drugs are helpful if there are concerns about adherence. The long duration of action gives a lasting antipsychotic effect but also means that any side effects are prolonged. A small test dose is administered at the start of treatment, which is increased slowly, and the absolute minimum dose necessary for symptom control is used.

Anxiolytics and hypnotics

Benzodiazepines

Mode of action

Benzodiazepines act at specific receptor sites on GABA-A receptors and enhance GABA neurotransmission. Changes in these receptors with age increase the sensitivity of older people to this group of drugs.

Indications

The use of benzodiazepines is avoided where possible because of the risk of sedation, confusion and falls. They are used mainly for the short-term management of acute anxiety and insomnia. Other indications include alcohol withdrawal, acute behavioural disturbances and epilepsy. Management of these disorders is discussed in the relevant chapters.

When benzodiazepines are prescribed there should be a plan for early review. Use should not normally continue for more than two to four weeks.

Temazepam and nitrazepam are commonly used as hypnotics. Drugs with longer half-lives (e.g. diazepam, see Table 10.39) can cause a hangover effect.

Table 10.39   Half-lives of benzodiazepines

Drug	Approximate half-life (hours)
Chlordiazepoxide	5–30 (active metabolite up to 200)
Clonazepam	20–40
Diazepam	20–70 (active metabolite up to 200)
Lorazepam	10–20
Nitrazepam	15–38
Oxazepam	4–15
Temazepam	8–22

Diazepam is the benzodiazepine most often used in the management of anxiety disorders. The initial effect of a single dose will wear off within a few hours. Regular administration leads to accumulation of its less active metabolite, which is slow to be eliminated, and leads to a more constant anxiolytic effect. Diazepam therefore carries an increased risk in older people because of the risk of accumulation leading to toxicity.

Lorazepam has a short half-life and rapid onset of action, and can be administered orally or intramuscularly. It is used relatively often in the management of acutely disturbed or anxious younger adults, but this use does not translate well into old age psychiatry where the risks of side effects usually outweigh potential benefit. The first dose should not exceed 0.5 mg.

Dosage

Older people are generally much more sensitive to benzodiazepines than younger people, and effective doses may be surprisingly low. 1 mg of diazepam can have a significant effect and it is important to start at low doses and titrate up if necessary. When used for hypnotic effect, a quarter to one half of the adult dose is usually adequate and more than this may be unsafe.

Side effects

Box 10.13   Side effects of benzodiazepines

Sedation

Confusion

Ataxia

Dizziness

Paradoxical agitation

Disinhibition

Respiratory depression (avoid in COPD)

Dependence

Older people are particularly vulnerable to the side effects of benzodiazepines (Box 10.13). Sedation, confusion and ataxia increase the risk of falls and elderly people who are prescribed benzodiazepines have a 50 % increased risk of fractured hip.

There is also a risk of respiratory depression, particularly with co-existing lung disease (Table 10.40). Side effects may not be immediately obvious and may become apparent after several days with accumulation of the drug or its active metabolite.

Table 10.40 Risks associated with benzodiazepine use in co-morbid illness

Condition	Comments
Respiratory disease, e.g. COPD	Risk of respiratory depression
Hepatic impairment	Active metabolites may accumulate, especially with diazepam Risk of precipitating hepatic encephalopathy
Renal impairment	Low dose lorazepam safest option but avoid if possible
Dementia	Risk of exacerbation of cognitive impairment

Interactions

The additive effects of other sedative drugs (including alcohol) can lead to dangerous levels of sedation and even fatal respiratory depression.

Tolerance, dependence and withdrawal

Tolerance and dependence will develop with long-term administration of benzodiazepines. Withdrawal symptoms can develop when a drug is abruptly stopped after as little as two weeks of administration (Box 10.14).

Box 10.14   Features of benzodiazepine withdrawal

Anxiety

Tremor

Dizziness

Nausea

Tinnitus

Sweating

Visual disturbances

Paraesthesiae

Depersonalisation

Use should ideally be limited to short periods but in practice many people are prescribed long-term benzodiazepines, sometimes for many years. In these cases it is

Table 10.41 Doses equivalent to 10 mg diazepam for other benzodiazepines

Drug	Dose equivalent to 10 mg diazepam
Chlordiazepoxide	25 mg
Clonazepam	1–2 mg
Lorazepam	1 mg
Nitrazepam	10 mg
Oxazepam	30 mg
Temazepam	20 mg

Source: Maudsley Prescribing Guidelines 2007

important to weigh up the risks and benefits to the patient of withdrawing treatment. If the patient is not sedated or experiencing falls or other side effects, the safest option may be to leave things as they are rather than risk withdrawal symptoms. When benzodiazepines are withdrawn, the drug is converted to the equivalent dose of diazepam (Table 10.41) and the dose is very slowly reduced, for example by 10 % of the daily dose every month.

Overdose

If a patient is given a dose of benzodiazepine that is too high the most serious complication is respiratory depression or arrest. If this occurs, the patient will need ventilatory support and emergency transfer to a medical unit. Principles of basic life support apply. Flumazenil can be given i.v. to reverse the effects of benzodiazepines but be aware that its half-life is shorter than that of diazepam and it has the potential to cause seizures.

Buspirone

Buspirone is a partial agonist at the 5-HT 1A receptor, licensed for short-term use in generalised anxiety disorder. The anxiolytic effect usually develops within two to four weeks; tolerance and dependence do not occur and there is no withdrawal syndrome. In the elderly it is probably less effective than the antidepressants used in the treatment of anxiety (page 95).

Common side effects include nausea, nervousness, light-headedness and headache. Confusion can occur but is unusual and buspirone does not have sedative properties. There is little potential for interaction although combination with MAOIs is avoided.

Pregabalin

Pregabalin is an antiepileptic drug that has recently been licensed for use in generalised anxiety disorder. Its short-term efficacy has been demonstrated in both younger adults and the elderly in placebo-controlled trials.

Side effects include sedation, constipation, dry mouth, dizziness, blurred vision, weight gain, oedema, muscle weakness and tremor. There appears to be a minimal effect on cognitive function that is much smaller than with the benzodiazepines. Tolerance and dependence do not develop but when stopping the dose must be gradually reduced to avoid withdrawal symptoms (insomnia, nausea, headache, diarrhoea).

Antidepressants

Many antidepressants are used in the management of anxiety disorders (see page 95). TCAs are sometimes prescribed for insomnia but in the absence of depression their use is not justified. Trazodone is also sometimes used in insomnia and has a safer side-effect profile than the TCAs but there is no evidence for its use in non-depressed patients.

Beta-blockers

Beta-blockers are sometimes used to treat the physiological symptoms of anxiety. Blocking peripheral β-adrenergic receptors reduces tremor, sweating, tachycardia and palpitations in younger patients but there is little evidence supporting the use of these drugs in the elderly. They can precipitate heart failure and are contraindicated in asthma and COPD. Diabetic patients who are taking beta-blockers are less able to recognise features of hypoglycaemia. Side effects are summarised in Box 10.15.

Box 10.15   Side effects of beta-blockers

Bradycardia

Hypotension

Bronchospasm

Heart failure

Peripheral vasoconstriction

Insomnia

Sexual dysfunction

Tiredness

Newer hypnotic drugs: zopiclone, zolpidem and zaleplon

Zopiclone, zolpidem and zaleplon ("Z" drugs) are structurally different from the benzodiazepines but act at or near to the benzodiazepine receptor site. They are indicated for use in the short-term management of insomnia. Tolerance and dependence occur and abruptly stopping the drug leads to a withdrawal syndrome similar to that seen with benzodiazepines.

Table 10.42 Dose, time to onset, half-life and effects of hypnotic drugs on sleep

Drug	Dose (mg)	Time to onset (minutes)	Half-life (hours)	⇓ Sleep latency	⇓ Night waking	⇓ REM sleep
Temazepam	10	30–60	8–22	✓	✓	✓
Nitrazepam	2.5–5	20–50	15–38	✓	✓	✓
Zopiclone	3.75	15–30	9*	✓	✓	×
Zaleplon	5	30	1	✓	?×	×
Zolpidem	5	7–27	3	✓	✓	×

*6 hours in the under 65s

Side effects and toxicity

The "Z" drugs are relatively safe in overdose and their effects are reversed by the benzodiazepine antagonist flumazenil. All can cause gastrointestinal disturbances, dizziness, confusion and falls. The most common side effect with zopiclone is a metallic taste. They may be just as likely as benzodiazepines to cause dependence and rebound insomnia.

NICE conclude that there is no compelling evidence to distinguish between zopiclone, zolpidem, zaleplon and the short-acting benzodiazepines. They advise that the least expensive drug is prescribed and if patients do not respond to one drug they should not be prescribed another.

Drugs used in dementia

Cholinesterase inhibitors

There is significant evidence that cholinesterase inhibitors are effective in Alzheimer's disease, dementia with Lewy bodies and vascular dementia. The strongest evidence is for mild to moderate Alzheimer's disease, where there is an initial modest improvement in cognition and a slower rate of cognitive decline with treatment. Cholinesterase inhibitors may also be helpful in treating behavioural and psychological symptoms of dementia and some studies have shown improvements in global functioning, activities of daily living and carer burden.

Cholinesterase inhibitors provide symptomatic improvements and do not target the underlying pathology of the disease; they cannot prevent eventual deterioration. At present, NICE guidelines (page 40) recommend the use of cholinesterase inhibitors only in moderate Alzheimer's disease.

The drugs available are donepezil, rivastigmine and galantamine. There is no clear evidence that any one is more effective than another although individual patients may tolerate the side effects of one drug better than others. A decision regarding clinical benefit and continuing treatment is made after three to six months.

Mechanism of action

Donepezil and galantamine are reversible inhibitors of acetylcholinesterase and galan-tamine also acts as an agonist at nicotinic receptors. Rivastigmine is a reversible non-competitive acetylcholinesterase inhibitor. All of these drugs increase the concentration of acetylcholine in the synaptic cleft and enhance cholinergic neurotransmission.

Dose and preparations

Table 10.43 Dose and preparations of cholinesterase inhibitors

Drug	Starting dose	Titration	Maintenance dose (mg/day)	Preparations available			
				Tab	Caps	Liq	Patch
Donepezil	5 mg once daily	↑ to 10 mg after one month if necessary	5–10	√	×	×	×
Rivastigmine	1.5 mg twice daily	↑ by 1.5 mg b.d. every four weeks as necessary	6–12	×	√	√	√
Galantamine	8 mg once daily*	↑ by 8 mg/day every four weeks as necessary	16–24	√	√	√	×

Caps = capsules Liq = liquid, oral solution or oral drops   Patch = dermal patch   *Modified release form (capsules), twice daily dosing form is available as a tablet

The starting dose is low and is titrated up according to tolerance and clinical response. Once-daily preparations are often a better choice if there are concerns about adherence although if medication is supervised this is less of an issue.

Side effects

Most side effects (Table 10.44) relate to cholinergic activity and many can be avoided by starting at a low dose that is gradually titrated up. If side effects occur, the dose can be

Table 10.44 Side effects of cholinesterase inhibitors

Gastrointestinal	Neurological	Cardiac	Respiratory
Nausea	Insomnia	Arrhythmias	Worsening of asthma or
Vomiting	Dizziness	Bradycardia	COPD
Diarrhoea	Headache	Heart block	
Anorexia	Tremor	*All patients need an ECG*	
Abdominal pain	Syncope	*before starting treatment*	
Weight loss	Muscle cramps		
Gastric/duodenal ulceration/haemorrhage	Seizures		

reduced and later increased more slowly. If this does not work, another cholinesterase inhibitor may be better tolerated.

Cardiac side effects   All patients must have an ECG before starting treatment with a cholinesterase inhibitor. Arrhythmias and first-degree heart block are not absolute contraindications, but it is wise to discuss the issue with a cardiologist.

Interactions

There is a relatively low potential for interactions; rivastigmine may be the least likely to interact with other drugs.

Memantine

There is evidence that memantine is effective in the treatment of moderate to severe Alzheimer's disease although current NICE guidelines support its use only within clinical research. It may have an additive effect when given together with a cholinesterase inhibitor. Like the cholinesterase inhibitors, it is a symptomatic treatment and does not affect the disease process.

Mode of action

Memantine is an N-methyl-D-aspartate (NMDA) receptor antagonist. Glutamate and the NMDA receptor play an important role in learning and memory under normal conditions. In Alzheimer's disease glutamate activity may be increased, leading to sustained activation of NMDA receptors and impairment of neuronal function. Memantine is believed to modify this activity without impairing the glutamate-mediated neurotransmission necessary for normal cognitive function.

Dose

The starting dose is 5 mg once daily, increased by 5 mg each week to a maximum of 10 mg b.d.

Side effects

Table 10.45 Side effects of memantine

Common	Unusual	Rare
Constipation	Vomiting	Seizures
Headache	Confusion	Pancreatitis
Dizziness	Fatigue	Psychosis
Drowsiness	Hallucinations	Depression
	Abnormal gait	

Interactions

Memantine has a higher potential for interaction than the cholinesterase inhibitors. Interactions include enhancement of the effects of anticholinergics, antipsychotics, selegiline and warfarin.

Other drugs

Many drugs and nutritional supplements have been investigated for use in the treatment of dementia, including:

- Antioxidants (gingko biloba, vitamin E and fish oils)

- Anti-inflammatory drugs

- Hormone replacement therapy.

However, evidence is generally weak or limited and at present none are recommended for the treatment or prevention of dementia.

Disease modifying treatments

Future treatments aimed at disease modification may target:

- Secretase pathways, to reduce production of β-amyloid

- Prevention of β-amyloid aggregation

- Vaccination with β-amyloid or antibodies against β-amyloid

- Tau and its phosphorylation.

Pharmacological treatment of behavioural and psychological symptoms of dementia (BPSD)

When drugs are used for the behavioural and psychiatric symptoms of dementia, it should be in the context of a management plan involving social, psychological and behavioural interventions. The evidence for pharmacological interventions is summarised in Table 10.46. Low doses are used, particularly with antipsychotic drugs. Doses of 0.5 mg haloperidol, 2.5 mg olanzapine or 0.5 mg risperidone may be adequate and starting doses should not be higher than this. See page 28 for further information about BPSD.

Table 10.46 Evidence for pharmacological interventions in the behavioural and psychiatric symptoms of dementia

Drug	Comments
Typical antipsychotics	Evidence for small improvement but high rate of side effects No difference between individual drugs shown
Atypical antipsychotics	Modest effects of risperidone and olanzapine shown Increased risk of stroke No trials of other atypicals but likely to have similar effects
Antidepressants	Only evidence is for citalopram, small effect size
Valproate	Several RCTs have shown no improvement More side effects than placebo, including sedation
Carbamazepine	Two small studies, one positive one negative
Cholinesterase inhibitors	Improvements shown, may not be clinically significant
Memantine	Conflicting results, possible effect
Benzodiazepines	Lorazepam is the only benzodiazepine studied Risk of tolerance, dependence, falls Not recommended, if used must be low dose and short-term

Source: Sink *et al.* (2005)

Further reading

BMA and RPS (2007) *The British National Formulary 54 (September 2007)* London, Pharmaceutical Press.

Bouman W and Pinner G (2002) Use of antipsychotic drugs in old age psychiatry *Adv Psych Treatment* 8: 49–58.

Burns A and O'Brien J (2006) Clinical practice with anti-dementia drugs: a consensus statement from British Association for Pharmacology *J Psychopharmacol* 20: 732–755.

Cookson J, Taylor D and Katona K (2002) *Use of Drugs in Psychiatry* London, Gaskell.

Cooper C, Carpenter IC, Katona C *et al.* (2005) The AdHOC study of older adults' adherence to medication in 11 countries *Am J Geriat Psychiat* 13: 1067–1076.

Cusack BJ (2004) Pharmacokinetics in older persons *Am J Geriat Pharmacother* 2: 274–302.

Greenberg RM and Kellner CH (2005) Electroconvulsive therapy: a selected review *Am J Geriat Psychiat* 13(4): 268–281.

Lléo A, Greenberg SM and Growdon JH (2006) Current pharmacotherapy for Alzheimer's disease *Annu Rev Med* 57: 513–533.

Katona C and Livingstone G (2003) *Drug Treatment in Old Age Psychiatry* London, Martin Dunitz.

Nabil S, Kamel MD and Gammack JK (2006) Insomnia in the elderly: cause, approach and treatment *Am J Med* 119: 463–469.

Roose SP and Schatzberg AF (2005) The efficacy of antidepressants in the treatment of late-life depression *J Clin Psychopharmacol* 25(4) Suppl 1: S1–S7.

Routledge PA, O'Mahony MS and Woodhouse KW (2004) Adverse drug reactions in elderly patients *Br J Clin Pharmacol* 57(2): 121–126.

Sink KM, Holden KF and Yaffe K (2005) Pharmacological treatment of neuropsychiatric symptoms of dementia *JAMA* 293: 596–608.

Taylor D, Paton C and Kerwen R (2007) *The South Maudsley Prescribing Guidelines (9th Edition)* London, Informa Healthcare.

Turnheim K (2004) Drug therapy in the elderly *Exp Gerontology* 39: 1731–1738.

11

Electroconvulsive Therapy

In electroconvulsive therapy (ECT), an electric current is used to induce a seizure whilst the patient is anaesthetised. ECT is one of the most effective means of treating severe depression in both younger and older adults, particularly when psychotic features are present. Perhaps unsurprisingly, it is also one of the most controversial treatments in psychiatry. It is therefore important to have an understanding of the indications, risks, benefits and practicalities of the procedure.

The Old Age Psychiatry Handbook   Joanne Rodda, Niall Boyce, and Zuzana Walker
© 2008 John Wiley & Sons, Ltd

Indications

The main indication for ECT is *severe depressive illness* in which there is life-threatening refusal of food or fluid, risk of suicide, or psychotic features. Other indications for ECT are summarised below. Guidelines from NICE (Box 11.1) and the Royal College of Psychiatrists (Table 11.1) differ somewhat.

Box 11.1   Indications for ECT: NICE guidance

Treatment resistant or potentially life-threatening:

– severe depressive illness

– catatonia

– prolonged or severe manic episode

These guidelines apply to the general adult population. Evidence also supports the use of ECT in depression in the elderly. There is little evidence to draw on regarding the use of ECT in mania and schizophrenia in the elderly.

Mechanism of action

The specific mode of action is unclear. ECT has wide ranging effects on neurotransmitters, receptors and the hypothalamo-pituitary-adrenal axis.

Table 11.1   Indications for ECT: Royal College of Psychiatrists

Depression	Treatment of choice in: – life-threatening refusal of food/fluid – high suicide risk Consider in depressive illness associated with: – severe psychomotor retardation/stupor – psychotic features – non-response to drug treatment
Mania	Life threatening physical exhaustion Failure of drug treatment
Schizophrenia	Fourth-line treatment after two antipsychotics and clozapine
Catatonia	If treatment with benzodiazepine has failed

Efficacy

Response rates for ECT in the treatment of depression in the elderly are reported to be in the range of 80–90 %. This figure falls to 50–60 % if ECT follows a period of ineffective pharmacological treatment. Response to ECT is also faster than response to antidepressants, and significant clinical improvement is usually evident within a few treatments.

Adverse effects

Following ECT, it is common for patients to experience loss of memory for periods of up to 30 minutes before (*retrograde amnesia*) and after (*anterograde amnesia*) the treatment. Less commonly, these deficits may be more extensive. There may also be a brief period of *disorientation* or *headache*.

Other adverse effects, like tongue or lip-biting or minor electrical burns from incorrect electrode placements, are avoided by using proper procedure.

Box 11.2   Adverse effects of ECT

Brief retrograde and anterograde amnesia

Brief disorientation

Headache

Muscle pains

Complications of anaesthesia

Unilateral ECT (electrodes are placed on one side of the skull only) may have a similar clinical effect but fewer adverse effects. However, there is no evidence to support the use of unilateral rather than bilateral ECT in the elderly.

The risks of anaesthesia are as for a minor surgical procedure; the reported mortality rate is 2 in 100 000. Older people are more likely to have co-morbid physical illness and may be at higher risk from anaesthesia.

Cautions

It is widely quoted that there are no absolute contraindications for ECT. However most clinicians would give ECT only in *extreme* circumstances where there is:

- Recent myocardial infarction

- Cardiac arrhythmias

- Recent stroke

- Raised intracranial pressure

- Cerebral or other vascular aneurysm

- Other conditions that increase anaesthetic risk.

    Dementia, Parkinson's disease and epilepsy are not contraindications for ECT.

Consent

Before informed consent can be given by the patient, the risks, benefits and procedure of ECT must be explained to them in a way that is easily understood. Information leaflets can be helpful, and time must be allowed for discussion with family or friends if required. Patients must be aware that they can withdraw consent at any time.

ECT and the Mental Health Act

If a patient detained under the Mental Health Act 1983 (England and Wales) does not consent or is unable to consent to ECT when it is seen as essential, a second opinion from an independent doctor must be sought.

Pre-ECT physical work-up

It is particularly important in elderly patients that appropriate investigations are completed before ECT. These include:

- Physical examination

- Full blood count

Table 11.2 Medication during ECT

Drug group	Comment
Benzodiazepines/hypnotics	Increase seizure threshold
	Avoided during ECT where possible
Anticonvulsants	Increase seizure threshold
	Continued during ECT
	May need higher stimulus dose
Antidepressants	Lower seizure threshold
	Continue during ECT
	Moclobemide is stopped 24 hours before ECT (anaesthetic risk)
	Discuss MAOIs with anaesthetist
Antipsychotics	Lower seizure threshold
	Continue during ECT
Acetylcholinesterase inhibitors	Discuss with anaesthetist

- Urea and electrolytes

- ECG

- Chest x-ray

- Any other investigations indicated by physical illnesses.

Medication and ECT

Many psychotropic medications increase or decrease the seizure threshold. Benzodiazepines and hypnotic drugs are avoided during a course of ECT where possible because they increase seizure threshold. Anticonvulsants, antipsychotics and antidepressants are usually continued where clinically indicated.

ECT procedure

The procedure for ECT will be different in different hospitals; a general checklist for ECT treatment is given in Box 11.3.

Box 11.3   Checklist for ECT treatment

Check patient ID

Check consent signed

Check patient has fasted and emptied bowels/bladder

Check monitoring attached (ECG, EEG, BP etc.)

After patient anaesthetised, ensure bite guard placed

Place electrodes (see local guidance)

Select stimulus according to local policy

Test contact, then deliver ECT

Record:

   – energy dose

   – visible seizure duration

   – EEG seizure duration

   – complications

Patient will recover in recovery room with nurse(s) and doctor(s) present

---

Seizure length

A visual seizure length of 20 seconds is said to be a marker of effective treatment. The "gold standard" for monitoring seizures is the EEG. The length of the seizure appearing on the EEG will be longer than the visual seizure, and is usually 35–130 seconds in length.

Energy dose

Ideally, the lowest energy dose that will cause a seizure of sufficient duration is used. Excess current above that required to cause a seizure will increase post-ECT memory loss and confusion. The method used to determine the energy dose will be set out in local policy. The dose required usually increases throughout a course of ECT, as ECT itself increases seizure threshold.

Stimulus dosing involves starting with a low dose and gradually increasing until a seizure occurs. During the following treatments the dose is then increased to two or three times the seizure threshold. In *age dosing* the dose is set according to predetermined levels for age. This is simpler but may result in higher doses than necessary being used.

Frequency and number of treatments

A course of ECT is usually between six and twelve sessions. ECT is usually twice weekly; no additional benefit has been shown from greater frequency.

Prevention of relapse

There is a high risk of relapse in the weeks following a successful course of ECT. Patients who have had ECT should continue with antidepressant treatment. In the elderly maintenance antidepressant treatment may need to be lifelong.

Further reading

Scott AIF (2005) College guidelines on electroconvulsive therapy: an update for prescribers *Adv Psychiat Treat* 11: 150–156.

Salzman C, Wong E and Wright BC (2002) Drug and ECT treatment of depression in the elderly 1996–2001: a literature review *Biol Psychiat* 52: 265–284.

Van Ser Wurff FB, Stek ML, Hoogendijk WL and Beekman ATF (2002) Electroconvulsive therapy for the depressed elderly *Cochrane Database Syst Rev* 2: CD 003593.

12

Psychological Therapies

There is a growing evidence base for the use of psychotherapeutic treatment in elderly patients. Besides the formal psychotherapies, innovative techniques have been developed for use in individuals with dementia.

Cognitive behavioural therapy

More emphasis has been placed on the explanation of CBT than other therapies, given its widespread use in clinical practice and the significant evidence base for its application in the elderly population.

Since its development in the 1960s, CBT has become one of the most widely used and influential psychological therapies. In younger adults, it has been shown to be effective in many psychiatric disorders, most notably depression and anxiety.

There is growing evidence for the effectiveness of CBT in elderly patients. Studies in this population also suggest a role for CBT in helping those with chronic illness or

The Old Age Psychiatry Handbook   Joanne Rodda, Niall Boyce, and Zuzana Walker
© 2008 John Wiley & Sons, Ltd

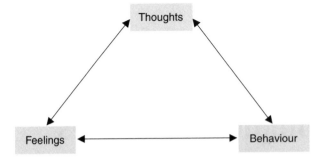

Figure 12.1 CBT is based on the principle that thoughts, feelings and behaviour are interrelated and modifiable

pain. Bibliotherapy (self-help literature) and remote-access CBT (using the internet) have been important advances in widening access to CBT for older patients who may have problems with mobility or transport.

CBT is often a brief intervention, consisting of 8 to 12 weekly sessions, either on an individual or group basis. However, therapy is tailored to the needs of the individual patient and some may benefit from a more prolonged period of treatment, sometimes several years. Sessions usually last around an hour and patients work collaboratively with their therapist. Key features of the therapeutic process include Socratic questioning (patients discover the truth for themselves) and regular homework tasks, which may include thought or activity diaries.

CBT is based on the concept that thoughts, feelings and behaviour are interrelated and, to an extent, modifiable (Figure 12.1). An example is a patient who is depressed and believes that no-one cares about them. One resulting behaviour may be that he avoids social contact, reinforcing his negative belief and further lowering mood: a vicious cycle. This problem can be approached by addressing behaviours (e.g. gradually increasing social activities) in addition to focusing on the nature, origin and influence of negative cognitions.

Depression and the CBT model

Early in childhood, people develop beliefs about themselves, the world and others (Beck's cognitive triad). These *core beliefs* or *core schemas* are held as absolute truths. Based on his or her core beliefs, an individual will develop "assumptions" or rules by which they believe they must live their life. This can be illustrated by considering a CBT model of depression (Figure 12.2).

Negative thinking patterns in depression are believed to emerge in early life. On the basis of adverse experiences, patients develop negative core schema. Using these schemas they devise erroneous guidelines for living known as "conditional dysfunctional assumptions", e.g. "I must be the best if I am to stay happy."

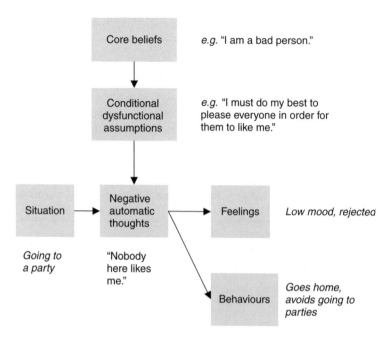

Figure 12.2   Outline of the CBT model and example

In a specific situation, these assumptions may be activated, leading to repetitive and unintentional *negative automatic thoughts*, e.g. "I'm no good at this." or "She doesn't like me." As outlined previously and in Figure 12.1, these negative automatic thoughts can affect feelings and behaviour, creating a vicious cycle.

One of the key concepts in CBT is that the impact of a given situation on the thoughts, feelings and behaviour of an individual will depend on their *perception* of that situation. This will be determined to a great extent by their unique core beliefs and assumptions.

Negative automatic thoughts, in turn, are maintained by a number of *cognitive distortions*. These are errors in thinking or perception that reinforce negative cognitions and have been shown to be more common during a depressive illness. Examples are given in Table 12.1.

Summary

CBT is an effective therapeutic strategy for a number of different psychiatric presentations in elderly patients. The therapist works actively with the patient to develop their understanding of the interactions between thoughts, feelings and behaviour and to identify and modify dysfunctional cognitive and behavioural patterns. Of particular

Table 12.1 Examples of cognitive distortions in depression

Example	Brief description
Arbitrary inference	Jumping to false conclusions
Selective abstraction	Seeing only the negative aspects of a situation
Dichotomous thinking	A situation is only viewed as one of two polarised possibilities, e.g. "If I am not perfect I am a complete failure."
Overgeneralisation	Sweeping negative generalisation based on a single situation
Personalisation	Negative behaviours in others are seen as related to the individual, e.g. "He is upset, I must have done something wrong."
Magnification/minimisation	Magnification of negative aspects whilst minimising positive aspects of a situation

relevance in older adults, a certain level of cognitive ability is needed to benefit from therapy. However, patients with dementia can still benefit from CBT tailored to their individual needs.

Behavioural therapy

Behavioural therapy is a brief, focused, practical intervention based on psychological learning theories. Using theories such as classical conditioning (Pavlov), operant conditioning (Gross) and social learning theory (Bandura) behavioural therapy seeks to encourage patients to learn though associations. In this way, maladaptive associations are "unlearned", resulting in a reduction in undesirable behaviours and/or an increase in more adaptive behaviours. Unlike in CBT, the changes resulting from behavioural therapy occur at a non-conscious level.

Behaviour therapy is often conducted indirectly by working with staff members or carers. This process often begins with a functional analysis of the behaviour in terms of the **a**ntecedents, **b**ehaviour and **c**onsequences (ABC). Individual factors associated with the behaviour are considered, as are the context and setting. In addition, an assessment of the patient's strengths and interests is often made in order to tailor rewards. Observation of the behaviour from witnesses or through diary accounts is important. The aim of the therapy is to modify any external factors that may be reinforcing the problematic behaviour. Reinforcement of more adaptive behaviours is simultaneously increased. RCT evidence exists for using this approach in managing behavioural difficulties in patients with dementia.

In other cases, the therapist works directly with the patient. With the therapist's guidance, the patient is able to identify and modify problematic behaviours. For example, in the case of phobias, therapy often involves graded exposure to the phobic stimulus. These techniques have largely been incorporated into cognitive behavioural therapy.

Psychoanalytic psychotherapy

Psychoanalytic psychotherapy has historically been seen as most suitable for a younger patient group. However, there is a growing consensus that a role exists for psychoanalytic psychotherapy in helping patients negotiate what could be defined as the final developmental process of life. As such, patients with mood disorders, anxiety disorders and/or personality difficulties may benefit from this form of therapy. The evidence base for this type of therapy has been difficult to establish but there is some relatively limited support for its use.

Psychoanalytic psychotherapy is based on the principle that unconscious mental processes are shaped by experiences in early relationships, and have a critical bearing on present difficulties, interactions and behaviour. These problems are often the result of unconscious internal conflicts or anxiety. Defence mechanisms are deployed to reduce these conflicts, which may in turn contribute to the current difficulties.

Psychoanalytic therapists adopt a non-directive approach, relying on their patients to use 'free association' to share any thoughts, dreams, or fantasies that may come to mind. The therapist listens and makes minimal responses, enabling the patient to project their internal object relations onto them. He or she seeks to make interpretations about the processes that occur within the patient's relationships, including their relationship with the therapist. The feelings of the patient towards the therapist (transference) and the feelings elicited in the therapist by the patient (countertransference) are particularly important. The aim of therapy is to improve the patient's insight and to lessen the need to use unhelpful defence mechanisms in response to their anxiety. Consistency in timing, location and duration of sessions and the therapist's interactions with the patient are crucial.

The practicalities of psychoanalytic psychotherapy may present challenges for older patients.

Box 12.1 Key requirements for psychodynamic psychotherapy

The patient must be able to:

- attend regular scheduled appointments (usually weekly) for a significant duration of time, often for two to three years

- think of their problems in psychological terms

- demonstrate insight and motivation for change

- demonstrate sufficient ego strength to withstand difficult feelings that may arise

- refrain from misuse of alcohol/illicit drugs

Patients must have sufficient ego strength to engage in psychoanalytic psychotherapy. Essentially, this refers to the capacity of the individual to not have to resort to defences that grossly impair their ability to be in touch with reality, or to very destructive defences (for example self-harm) when they are faced with psychological distress.

Sometimes psychoanalytic therapy can be difficult to access or some patients may find it difficult to tolerate. For these patients, other forms of psychodynamic psychotherapy may be available that adopt a more flexible and supportive approach.

Family therapy

There is increasing support for the role of family therapy in the elderly. There are three main family therapy schools. *Structural therapists* emphasise the importance of hierarchies and challenge dysfunctional alliances and inadequate or rigid boundaries. *Strategic therapists* view presenting problems in terms of dysfunctional patterns of communication and suggest symptoms may be a means of exerting control in relationships. *Systemic theorists* further developed the principles of the earlier schools and systemic therapy is now the most widely used form of therapy. It is based on the principle that every part of the family system has an impact on every other part of the system. Systemic therapists help the family to explore the interactions and beliefs within the family system.

Interpersonal psychotherapy

Interpersonal psychotherapy (IPT) is a structured, brief (usually 12 to 16 sessions) therapy. It is primarily used in the treatment of depression but may also be effective in other disorders, including bulimia nervosa. IPT does not view interpersonal difficulties as the only cause of depression but emphasises the principle that depression occurs within an interpersonal context.

The patient's problems are understood by reference to situations that arise in one or more of four interpersonal areas:

- Grief

- Interpersonal disputes (arguments, disagreements and disappointments)

- Role transitions (e.g. retirement)

- Interpersonal sensitivity (difficulties in establishing/maintaining supportive relationships).

The therapist and patient work collaboratively. The focus of therapy is on the identification and modification of problems within current interpersonal relationships rather than the patient's underlying beliefs or enduring personality characteristics. Towards the end of therapy the focus moves towards identifying therapeutic gains and ways of anticipating and preventing similar problems in the future.

Other therapies

Patients with dementia may lack the cognitive skills necessary to benefit from the therapies that have been summarised so far, and so techniques geared specifically towards such patients have been developed.

Reality orientation therapy may be informal (consistent reorientation of the patient to time, place and person) or formal (in specific sessions with a therapist). Whilst evidence exists for its efficacy as a specific therapy in promoting social and intellectual function, many now consider it as one part of a general level of social and intellectual stimulation desirable in patients with dementia. There is some evidence that reality orientation therapy enhances the beneficial effect of anticholinesterase medication on cognition.

Validation therapy involves empathetic and supportive patient contact with verbal and non-verbal expression of support. There is little evidence for its efficacy in improving outcomes or objective measures of well-being for patients with dementia, but it is evidently desirable for staff to implement its principles of treating the individual patient as unique and valuable.

Reminiscence therapy aims to improve behaviour and cognition through promoting socialisation and intellectual stimulation. It involves regular patient meetings to discuss the past, often with audiovisual aids. The diversity of methods of reminiscence therapy partially explains the lack of a substantial evidence base for this treatment.

Further reading

Beck JS (1995) *Cognitive Therapy: Basics and Beyond* New York, Guildford Press.

Valenstein AF (2000) The older patient in psychoanalysis *J Am Psychoan Ass* 48: 1563–1589.

Cuijpers P, van Straten A and Smit F (2006) Psychological treatment of late-life depression: a meta-analysis of randomised controlled trials *Int J Geriat Psychiat* 21: 1139–1149.

Spector A, Thorgrimsen L, Woods B *et al.* (2003) Efficacy of an evidence-based cognitive stimulation therapy programme for people with dementia *Br J Psychiat* 183: 248–254.

Onder G, Zanetti O, Giacobini E *et al.* (2005) Reality orientation therapy combined with cholinesterase inhibitors in Alzheimer's disease: randomised controlled trial *Br J Psychiat* 187: 450–455.

Neal M and Barton Wright P (2003) Validation therapy for dementia *Cochrane Database Syst Rev* 3: CD001394.

Woods B, Spector A, Jones C, Orrell M and Davies S (2005) Reminiscence therapy for dementia *Cochrane Database Syst Rev* 2: CD001120.

13

Practical, Legal and Social Issues

There are many legal, social and ethical issues that are of particular relevance in old age psychiatry. An understanding of these issues by all healthcare professionals facilitates holistic care and improves multidisciplinary working.

This chapter covers:

- Provision of services

- Legal issues in old age psychiatry

- Social and financial issues in old age

Mental health law and provision of social services varies between regions and countries. The information in this chapter is most relevant to England and Wales, although similar systems operate in Scotland and Northern Ireland.

The Old Age Psychiatry Handbook   Joanne Rodda, Niall Boyce, and Zuzana Walker
© 2008 John Wiley & Sons, Ltd

Provision of services

Multidisciplinary working

Multidisciplinary working is central to the philosophy of care in old age psychiatry. Whilst each member of the team has their own specific role (see Table 13.1), there is a great deal of overlap. Any member of the team may be responsible for the coordination of a patient's care.

Table 13.1 Roles and responsibilities of members of the multidisciplinary team in old age psychiatry. Depending on the nature of the team, there may be additional members, for example physiotherapists and speech and language therapists

Team member	Role
Consultant and junior doctors	Assessment and clinical care of patients including pharmacological and non-pharmacological interventions. Care of both medical and psychiatric needs, including liaison with other medical teams.
In-patient psychiatric nurse	Assessment and nursing care of psychiatric inpatients. Provision of a therapeutic ward environment in close collaboration with all members of the multidisciplinary team.
Community psychiatric nurse (CPT)	Often a first point of contact for patients and carers. Diverse responsibilities may include ensuring the general well-being of patients and their carers in the community, coordination of services, monitoring of medication, organisation of social care packages and liaison with care homes.
Clinical psychologist	Draw on a range of different psychological approaches to develop a formulation of the patient's problems and to provide psychological interventions tailored to individual patient needs. Assist the multidisciplinary team in considering the psychological aspects of the patient's difficulties and their management. May also undertake neuropsychological assessments.
Occupational therapist (OT)	Aim to maximise level of functioning and independence in daily living skills, leisure, work and relationships. This is achieved through the use of specific activities, adaptation of the physical environment, graded treatment programmes and close collaboration with carers and other professionals and agencies.
Social worker	Assist patients with social aspects of their lives, for example care packages, financial needs (including benefits), accommodation and access to facilities such as day centres, lunch clubs etc. Often involved in general support and coordination of care, including carer's needs.

Box 13.1 Stages of the Care Programme Approach

Assessment of the patient's healthcare and social needs.

Collaboration of the multidisciplinary team, the patient, and their informal carers to create a care plan.

Appointment of a key worker (who may be any member of the professional team) to oversee the implementation of the care plan and act as the first point of contact for the patient.

Regular meetings to update the care plan.

Teams usually meet regularly and the efficiency of working will depend to a great extent on good communication between members. Important aspects of work within the team that are not mentioned in Table 13.1 include training, research, audit and management.

The Care Programme Approach

The Care Programme Approach (CPA) was introduced in 1991 as a framework for systematic discharge planning for inpatients, and optimal care of psychiatric patients in the community. The CPA operates in four stages.

The level at which the CPA operates depends on the needs of the patient.

Box 13.2 Levels of operation of the Care Plan Approach

Minimal CPA is implemented for relatively stable patients who will normally only require input from one team member.

More complex CPA is appropriate for less stable patients who require more support and continuing assessment by more than one member of the team.

Full (Enhanced) CPA is for patients who have severe, unstable mental illness that carries elements of risk to themselves and others.

The supervision register is used for patients at-risk to guarantee systematic and regular follow-up.

The Community Mental Health Team

The community mental health team (CMHT) exists to coordinate community care of patients, and is normally the first point of contact for referrals, which may come from a number of different sources. In general, referrals will be discussed in regular multidisciplinary meetings. The most appropriate member of the team will complete an initial assessment and may then request input from other professionals.

Day hospitals and day centres

Patients who require continuing assessment and input may be referred to day hospitals. The day hospital is staffed by mental health nurses and usually has input from one or more of the psychiatrists from the CMHT. Its functions include:

Box 13.3   Functions of the day hospital

Monitoring of the mental state, general well-being and level of function of patients.

Initiation and monitoring of medication (e.g. cholinesterase inhibitors).

Therapeutic activities, socialisation and psychological treatment.

Patients normally attend day hospitals on one or more days a week for several months or, in some cases, years.

Day centres allow structured therapeutic activities, but without medical input.

Acute hospital wards

Patients with acute mental health problems, who cannot be safely managed in the community, are admitted to acute inpatient care. Admissions to the acute ward may also be appropriate in certain other circumstances, for example to commence medication that will need close monitoring in the initial stages.

Continuing care

The funding for the ongoing care of elderly people can be a controversial area. In some circumstances in the UK, ongoing care is provided by NHS Continuing Care Units (CCUs). These units provide care for patients with continuing health (rather than social) needs and include specialist dementia units. Patients with dementia whose needs are too complex for nursing home or residential accommodation (for example severe behavioural symptoms and/or medical needs) may require this type of care. These patients require a high level of therapeutic input and supervision. Such admissions are generally for a long period whilst behavioural and medical interventions are implemented. In reality, local policy varies.

Legal issues in old age psychiatry

Knowledge of mental health law is essential for the practice of psychiatry. The following section summarises the essential aspects of English law with regard to old age psychiatry. English law also has jurisdiction in Wales. Similar principles exist in Scottish and Northern Irish law.

The Mental Health Act (MHA) 1983

Under the Mental Health Act 1983, patients with a *mental illness of a nature and degree* that warrants detention in hospital can be compulsorily admitted in situations where:

- There is a risk to others.

- There is a risk to self (this can include the risk of exploitation or provoked assault by others, as well as self-harm and suicide).

- There is a serious risk of deterioration in the patient's mental health if they do not accept admission and treatment.

The MHA specifically states that it cannot be used "by reason only of promiscuity or other immoral conduct, sexual deviancy or dependency on alcohol or drugs."

Important sections of the Mental Health Act are summarised in Table 13.2.

Appeals

A patient who is detained under the Mental Health Act may appeal to:

- *The Trust Managers*. The appeal will be heard at a *Managers' Hearing* by a panel of three hospital managers, who are independent of the medical team. The MHA code of practice states that a Managers' Hearing must be held when

  - the patient applies for discharge

  - the section is renewed by the Responsible Medical Officer (RMO)

  - the patient's nearest relative wishes to exercise their right to discharge the patient, and a report barring discharge has been filed by the RMO.

- *The Mental Health Review Tribunal (MHRT)*, a panel consisting of a layperson, a lawyer and an independent psychiatrist.

Table 13.2 The Mental Health Act

Section	Purpose	Location	Application	Medical recommendation	Duration	Right of appeal	Notes
2	Assessment	Community or ward	Nearest relative or approved social worker (ASW)	Two doctors, one must be approved under Section 12 MHA	28 days	Patient eligible to appeal to Mental Health Review Tribunal (MHRT) within 14 days	Used on evidence of mental disorder: "mental illness, arrested or incomplete development of mind, psychopathic disorder and any other disorder or disability of mind" (Section 1 MHA)
3	Treatment	Community or ward	As for Section 2		6 months	Patient eligible to appeal within first and second 6 months and subsequently annually	May follow on from Section 2 or Section 5(2) In cases of mental impairment/psychopathic disorder, treatment must be likely to alleviate condition/prevent deterioration
						MHRT mandatory every 3 years	
4	Admission for assessment	Community	Nearest relative or ASW	Any doctor	72 hours		Used when need for assessment is urgent

Section	Purpose	Location	Applicant	Duration	Outcome	Notes
5(2)	Emergency detention on ward	Ward	Doctor in charge of patient's care (includes junior doctors not on Section 12 register)	72 hours	Patient subsequently assessed by consultant and decision made on stopping section or requesting assessment for Sections 2/3	Ensure correct patient and trust details on form Specific diagnosis not necessary for form, but reasons for detention must be given *Never* prepare 5(2) forms "just in case"
5(4)	Emergency detention on ward	Ward	Registered mental health nurse or registered nurse for mental handicap	6 hours	Medical assessment follows	No medical recommendation required for section
136	Removal to a place of safety for assessment	Public place	Police officer	72 hours	Medical assessment follows	Places of safety include police stations and A&E units Once patient has been accepted by place of safety, police officer has no legal obligation to stay
135	Removal to a place of safety for assessment	Patient's home	Local magistrates	72 hours	Medical assessment follows	Allows police to force entry into patient's house and remove to place of safety

(Continued)

Table 13.2 (*Continued*)

Section	Purpose	Location	Application	Medical recommendation	Duration	Right of appeal	Notes
7	Guardianship under appointment from local authority	Community	ASW	Two doctors, one must be approved under Section 12 MHA	6 months initially	Patient may appeal within first 6 months	Guardian (normally senior social worker or relative) has powers to – require patient to reside at a specified place – require patient to attend specified place for medical treatment, occupation, education, training – require access to be given to the patient by a doctor, ASW or other specified person
25 (Patients in the Community Act 1995)	Supervised discharge	Community	Initiated by patient's consultant, must be approved by patient's GP and ASW		Open-ended	Patient or relative may appeal to MHRT	Supervisor (CPN, ASW, doctor) has power to convey patient to place of safety or treatment, but not to force entry into house Section 3 MHA must be used if patient is to be treated without consent at place of safety

---

Box 13.4 Preparing a report for an appeal hearing

The report begins with the patient's details and diagnosis.

This is followed by a summary of the patient's admission, details of the rationale for their section, and relevant past psychiatric and medical history including a brief outline of previous admissions /detentions under section.

The second half of the report brings the appeal board up to date with the continuing grounds for detention. One approach is to subdivide the report into the four areas: *nature and degree of illness, risk to self, risk to others, risk to health*, and to give dated evidence from the notes in support of each point. This is, as far as possible, a purely factual list of dates and events without subjective commentary.

Finally, the relevant facts should be summarised along with a brief outline of the rationale for continued detention and the current treatment plan.

Any part of the report that the mental health team agrees may be harmful for the patient to read is clearly marked. The rationale for non-disclosure is submitted to the panel in an attached document.

The report is clearly signed with the author's name, position and the date.

Under current legislation, the MHRT must discharge the patient from section unless the detaining authority can provide satisfactory evidence that continued detention is necessary.

Section 117 aftercare

When a patient has been detained under Section 3 of the MHA, the health care professionals and health authority have a specific duty to provide suitable aftercare. Section 117 effectively formalises this aspect of good practice and makes the patient eligible for funding for certain types of placement. If the patient is stable after a reasonable period of time, the Section 117 can be rescinded by the responsible clinician.

Physical illness

The Mental Health Act cannot be used to compel a patient to receive physical treatment against their will. A patient who is detained under the mental health act may still have capacity to refuse medical treatment for a physical illness. The temporary nature of delirium means that the majority of clinicians would consider the use of the Mental Capacity Act 2005, rather than the MHA, to be appropriate in detaining and treating such patients.

Box 13.5   The Bournewood Case

The Bournewood Case raised important issues with regard to the management of patients lacking mental capacity.

Mr HL, a 48 year-old man with autism, had been living with Mr and Mrs E, a couple who had treated him as "one of the family" since his discharge from Bournewood Hospital, Surrey in 1994. In July 1997, Mr HL's agitated behaviour at a day centre led to his informal re-admission to Bournewood. Whilst HL had not actively consented to his hospital admission, neither did he appear to be actively dissenting.

Nevertheless, Mr and Mrs E objected to this admission.

The case was eventually heard by the European Court of Human Rights, who ruled in favour of Mr and Mrs E on the grounds of Article 5 of the European Charter of Human Rights, the 'right to liberty'. This effectively equates an informal admission of patients such as Mr HL with a 'detention'.

This ruling implies that all patients who do not actively consent to their admission are being detained illegally. The logical conclusion is that the large number of informal inpatients with dementia who lack capacity should in fact be formally detained under the MHA. The ethical and practical implications of this decision are vast. It remains to be seen if a revision of the MHA will settle this issue.

'Diogenes syndrome'

'Diogenes syndrome' is an umbrella term used to describe the process by which some elderly people, by hoarding objects and neglecting cleanliness, come to live in a state of squalor. This may be due to an identifiable mental illness or impairment such as dementia or depression. However, in many cases, no mental health problems can be identified. In such cases, use of the Mental Health Act is inappropriate. A general practitioner is able to use Section 47 of the National Assistance Act 1948 in cases when it is felt the house poses a public health hazard – for example if it is demonstrated that the state of the house is attracting vermin. This act allows the person to be removed from his or her home, with no right of appeal. In such cases it is best to consult with the Public Health Officers from the local council.

Mental capacity – the Mental Capacity Act (MCA) 2005

The Mental Capacity Act 2005 became law in England and Wales in 2007. Its aims are:

- To protect the vulnerable who are not able to make their own decisions.

- To clarify who can take decisions, in which situations, and to set out the best procedure for this.

- To enable people to plan ahead for a time when they may lose capacity.

Similar legislation exists in Scotland (the Adults With Incapacity Act 2000).

Principles of the MCA

The MCA empowers patients by making an *assumption of capacity until proven otherwise*. The guiding principles are listed in Box 13.6. The act specifically states that it does not authorise anyone to give a patient treatment for a mental disorder, or to consent to a patient being given such treatment. The Mental Health Act 1983 continues to cover these eventualities.

Box 13.6   Guiding principles of the Mental Capacity Act 2005

A person must be assumed to have capacity unless it is established that he lacks capacity.

A person is not to be treated as unable to make a decision unless all practicable steps to help him to do so have been taken without success.

A person is not to be treated as unable to make a decision merely because he makes an unwise decision.

The powers of the act must be used only to support actions or decisions that are:

1. In the best interests of the individual concerned

2. As unrestrictive as possible of the individual's rights and freedom of action.

Paragraphs 44 (1–3) define a new criminal offence of *neglect*. It applies to individuals who may be carers, holders of Enduring or Lasting Power of Attorney, or court-appointed deputies. If these individuals are found guilty of ill-treatment or wilful neglect of the person in their care who lacks capacity, they can be fined, imprisoned for up to five years or both.

Judging capacity

The Code of Practice of the MCA defines the circumstances in which a specialist assessment of capacity is necessary by a medical expert such as an Old Age Psychiatrist. In other circumstances, a non-medical "lay" opinion is valid.

Box 13.7   Situations requiring specialist input when judging capacity

The decision and/or its consequences are grave.

The person concerned disputes a finding of incapacity.

There is disagreement between family members, carers and/or professionals as to the person's capacity.

A conflict of interest exists between the assessor and the person being assessed.

The person concerned is expressing different views to different people, perhaps through trying to please each or tell them what s/he thinks they want to hear.

The person's capacity to make a particular decision may be subject to challenge, either at the time the decision is made or in the future – for example, a will.

A vulnerable adult may lack capacity to make decisions that protect them against abuse.

The person concerned is repeatedly making decisions that put him/her at risk or resulting in preventable suffering or damage.

The person being assessed is involved in litigation, whether as plaintiff or defendant. In some cases the recommendation may follow that the assistance of the Official Solicitor or another "litigation friend" is required.

The finding of capacity has legal consequences (for example, a decision on compensation following a personal injury claim).

An assessment of capacity relates to a specific decision. A patient found not to have capacity to make the decision in question may still have capacity to make other decisions.

For both lay people and professionals, the criteria to determine capacity are the same. The individual is held to have capacity with regard to a decision if they can fulfil the criteria in Box 13.8.

If the person refuses an assessment, they should be advised regarding the consequences of this refusal (i.e. that their decisions will be open to challenge in future). However, it is generally agreed that it is not possible to force a capacity assessment on anyone. Many hospital trusts have introduced standardised forms to document the outcome of the capacity assessment.

Advance directives

Advance directives may be written or made orally. They are decisions made by competent individuals about which treatments they would want to be withheld or withdrawn in the event that they lose capacity.

The decision must be specific as to the exact treatment that would be refused. The individual may also describe the circumstances in which they envisage the refusal applying.

Box 13.8   Criteria for capacity with regard to a decision

To have capacity, a person must be able to:

– *Understand* the information relevant to the decision. The information must be given in a form that is appropriate to the patient's circumstances, such as "simple language, visual aids or any other means". The information given must include the reasonably foreseeable consequences of deciding one way or the other, and of failing to make the decision.

– *Retain* that information. The act stresses that if "a person is able to retain the information relevant to a decision for a short period only", it "does not prevent him from being regarded as able to make the decision."

– *Use or weigh* that information as part of the process of making the decision.

– *Communicate* his decision (whether by talking, using sign language or any other means).

Theoretically, if a patient subsequently finds him or herself in these circumstances, and lacks capacity, their decision is binding. However, the clinician can decide to go against an advance directive if he or she feels that:

• The decision was made under duress.

• The patient may not have been competent at the time of the directive.

• There are doubts about the patient's intentions.

• There are doubts as to whether or not the directive is valid (for example, a suicide note does not count as an advance directive).

The advice of relatives can be sought in making this decision. However, the MCA does not (and cannot) answer the question of whether the patient has accurately predicted how they will feel about treatment decisions in the future.

Lasting Power of Attorney

The MCA introduces the Lasting Power of Attorney. In contrast to the old Enduring Power of Attorney, which allowed a nominated person or persons to look after the property and financial affairs of another, the person given Lasting Power of Attorney (the LPA) may also make decisions on health and welfare issues for an individual who has lost capacity.

This power is, however, limited by several considerations. The LPA must believe that the person in their care lacks capacity, that action is necessary to prevent harm, and that this action is a proportionate response to the likelihood and seriousness of harm.

This effectively means that in circumstances when an individual lacks capacity, the doctor must ask the LPA for consent to treatment.

Doctors, particularly old age psychiatrists, will be asked to give an opinion on whether or not a patient is capable of making a Lasting Power of Attorney. This judgement should be made using similar principles to those governing testamentary capacity (see 'Wills', below). The 'donor' of the LPA should understand that they are signing an order which can only be revoked by the Court of Protection, that they are giving complete control of their property and potentially their life over to another person, and that this power will be conferred when they, the donor, lose capacity.

Changes to the Court of Protection

The creation of the LPA extended the role of the Court of Protection, which now deals with health and welfare as well as financial issues (see below). It has the power to appoint a deputy who will have ongoing powers to make decisions regarding patient care. However, this deputy is not able to refuse consent for life-sustaining treatment.

Research trials

The MCA allows "intrusive" research (which in a competent person would require consent) to be carried out on patients who lack capacity, provided that certain criteria are met:

Box 13.9 MCA criteria for intrusive research

This research either:

−has the potential to benefit the patient without imposing a burden that is dispro-
 portionate to the potential benefit

or

−is intended to provide knowledge of the causes or treatment of, or of the care of
 persons affected by, the same or a similar condition

In the latter case, when the research does not directly benefit the patient, the risk of harm must be negligible and the research must not interfere with the patient's freedom of action or privacy or be unduly invasive or restrictive.

Where possible, consultation with a relative is essential, and the likely wishes of the patient (if they still had capacity and were able to decide for themselves) must be taken into account.

Clinical trials are still covered by the Medicines for Human Use (Clinical Trials) Regulations 2004.

Independent mental capacity advocates

The MCA introduced an independent advocacy scheme to support those who lack capacity to make decisions. If there is no appropriate family member, friend, deputy or attorney and a decision must be made regarding placement or serious medical treatment, the independent advocate is asked to assist.

Consent to treatment

If the patient refuses treatment and has capacity to make their decision (see page 230), treatment cannot be given even if the consequences are likely to be fatal. If a patient undergoes a medical procedure without consent, the doctor may be liable for a charge of assault.

In patients who lack capacity, physical treatment can be given under the Mental Capacity Act. In such cases, a psychiatric opinion on capacity is necessary, and treatment must be in the best interests of the patient.

Box 13.10 Treatment in best interests

Treatment accepted by a majority of responsible medical practitioners

Treatment that is life-saving, or will ensure improvement/prevent deterioration in health

---

Prior to the introduction of the Mental Capacity Act, there was no legal basis for relatives' views to determine treatment. However, individuals appointed with Lasting Power of Attorney now have the right to make decisions on treatment of behalf of an incapacitated patient, with certain restrictions (see page 233).

The Code of Practice also advises that the lawfulness of certain treatments should be decided in court.

Withdrawing or withholding nutrition and hydration

Besides medical and surgical procedures, it is widely agreed that "treatment" also includes nasogastric, percutaneous or intravenous artificial nutrition and hydration (ANH).

Box 13.11   Court decisions of lawfulness of treatment

For the elderly, such decisions may include:

−withdrawing or withholding artificial nutrition and hydration from patients *in a persistent vegetative state*

−organ or bone marrow donation by a person without capacity

−dispute regarding what constitutes the patient's best interests

−ethical dilemmas in untested areas

Medical practitioners generally agree that ANH is subject to the same principles covered by consent to treatment.

In the case of patients with dementia, there is no evidence that nasogastric or percutaneous tube feeding improves survival or patient comfort, and it carries many risks (Box 13.12).

Box 13.12   Risks of artificial nutrition and hydration

Need for physical restraint to avoid patient removal of tube

Aspiration pneumonia

Diarrhoea/gastrointestinal discomfort

In renal failure, increased oral and pulmonary secretions lead to choking, dyspnoea and ascites

---

Some people may object to the withdrawal of ANH on an ethical and/or religious basis. Decisions on ANH can take these considerations into account, but must ultimately be made on the basis of the patient's best interests.

Financial issues

The Court of Protection

Prior to the introduction of the Mental Capacity Act 2005, the Court of Protection dealt solely with individuals who had lost the capacity to manage their finances.

If the patient has not set up a Lasting or Enduring Power of Attorney, the Court of Protection has the power to appoint a receiver to manage the patient's finances. This receiver may be a family member (who may make an application to the Court) or a professional. Non-professional receivers will not receive payment for their work.

The Court of Protection scrutinises the receiver's handling of the patient's finances. Usually it will require the receiver to supply a sum of money as security and to provide regular accounts.

Enduring Power of Attorney

In the past, the Enduring Power of Attorney allowed an individual (the donor) to nominate others to manage their financial affairs, should the donor lose capacity. This device has now been superseded by the Lasting Power of Attorney brought in by the Mental Capacity Act 2005 (see above).

Wills

Doctors, especially old age psychiatrists, are often asked to pass judgement on a patient's capacity to make a valid will ('testamentary capacity'). Disputed wills are costly to take to court, and cases in which the expenses of the case exceed the value of the will are not uncommon. Wills may appear frivolous or malicious, but if the patient has capacity, they are legally valid.

The basis of testamentary capacity in English Law was established by the Banks v Goodfellow case of 1870. The principles are listed in Box 13.13.

Box 13.13   Principles of testamentary capacity

A testator shall:

− understand the nature of its act and its effects

− understand the extent of the property of which (s)he is disposing

− be able to comprehend and appreciate the claims of those included and excluded by the will

− be unaffected by any mental disorder when considering the above

− not be under undue pressure from others when considering the above

---

It is not necessary for the testator to know the exact value of their assets, but they should have an overall idea of the form and proportion of these assets. It is important to explore the reasons as to why particular individuals are being included or excluded from the will, and to be satisfied that features of mental illness such as paranoia are not behind these decisions. In order to exclude the possibility of pressure from others, it is advisable to discuss the will in the absence of relatives or other interested parties.

Driving

Patients may still be driving when it is not safe for them to do so, for example due to mental illness, dementia or the effects of psychotropic drugs. It is essential to ask patients about driving, and to advise them accordingly. Guidelines for UK drivers are summarised in Table 13.3.

Social and financial issues in old age

Financial support

There are numerous sources of financial support for the elderly in the UK in addition to the basic state pension. It is useful to have a working knowledge of what options are available to patients.

The following section is intended as a basic outline of the options available in England and Wales. We have excluded schemes that are generally not available to retired people (e.g. Jobseeker's Allowance). Specific financial criteria have largely been omitted as these are subject to change. For up-to-date information, visit the Government's public services website (www.direct.gov.uk), the Age Concern website (www.ageconcern.co.uk), or contact your local authority or Citizens Advice Bureau.

Pensions

The *basic state pension* is paid from age 60 in women and age 65 in men. To qualify, a person must have paid or been credited with a sufficient number of National Insurance contributions.

Between 2010 and 2020 it is planned that the retirement age for men and women will be equalised.

The basic pension may be supplemented by a *private pension*, the *Pension Credit Scheme*, the *Industrial Injuries Scheme*, and *bereavement benefits*.

War widows or ex-servicemen and women who received injuries whilst in the armed forces can claim a *War Pension*.

Other benefits are summarised in Table 13.4.

Table 13.3 Guidelines for UK drivers

Condition	Guidelines
Minor, short-lived mental illness	No need for patient or the doctor to inform the Driver and Vehicle Licensing Authority (DVLA).
Severe anxiety and/or depression	Driving should cease pending further investigation. Period during which the patient cannot drive is decided on a case-by-case basis. DVLA are specifically concerned about those who may attempt suicide at the wheel.
Relapsing and remitting psychotic illness	Patient must not drive during the acute phase of the illness. After a 3-month period of stability, if the patient is compliant with treatment and the consultant offers a favourable report, driving licence will be reissued. The DVLA reserves the right to withhold the licence for longer if a patient has shown marked instability. The effect of medication on driving ability will also be taken into account.
Chronic symptoms of mental illness	DVLA will make a judgement as to how much these affect the ability to drive.
Alcohol misuse	Driving licence is likely to be suspended until a minimum of six months' abstinence has been achieved. In alcohol dependency, this period is extended to one year. If a patient experiences an alcohol-related seizure they must abstain from driving for one year. If the patient has an alcohol-related neuropsychiatric disorder (e.g. alcohol-related psychosis), licence will be revoked until satisfactory recovery is achieved.
Substance misuse	Misuse of cannabis, amphetamines, ecstasy and LSD will result in driving licence being suspended until the patient has been abstinent for six months. In the case of opiates, a one-year drug-free period is required, but patients on opiate substitutes such as methadone may be licensed. Those who misuse benzodiazepines must have been abstinent for one year before their licence will be re-issued.
Dementia	Patient must inform the DVLA. Licence will *not* be automatically revoked. In mild cases, licence may be issued subject to annual review. If the patient refuses to inform the DVLA, and as a clinician you have any concerns about the safety of others, *you* should inform the DVLA and inform the patient that you are doing so.

Table 13.4 UK benefits

Housing Benefit	Housing Benefit is provided to help those on low incomes to pay their rent. Alternatively, some local authorities contribute to rent for sheltered accommodation through "Supporting People" payments.
Council Tax	Properties *exempt* from Council Tax include "Granny Annexes" inhabited by an elderly relative, empty properties in which the owner is in a care home, and properties in which the liable occupant is "severely mentally impaired". If the property has features that are important for a disabled occupant (for example, space for a wheelchair), a *disability reduction* may be granted. *Discounts* are given if the house has only a single occupant, or if one of the occupants is a person with "severe mental impairment" or a carer. *Council Tax Benefits* are also available to help those who have difficulty paying due to low income.
Prescription charges and healthcare	Prescriptions are free for all people over the age of 60. NHS hearing aids and batteries are given on free loan. The cost of other items such as glasses, fabric supports etc. are dependent on income. Dental treatment is free for those on the Pension Credit Scheme, and free check-ups are available for people in Wales aged 60 and over.
TV licence	The UK TV licence is free for people over the age of 75. A reduction of 50 % is available for those registered as blind. Cheap concessionary licences are available for people who live in care homes or other eligible housing.
Telephone service	Some local authorities offer financial assistance with telephone line rental charges.
Utilities	A *Winter Fuel Payment* is made annually by the government to all people aged 60 and over. Those on the Pension Credit Scheme may receive additional *Cold Weather Payments*. The *Warm Front* scheme can provide a package of home heating improvements for those aged 60 and over on Pension Credit, Council Tax Benefits or Housing Benefits. Others can receive a *Heating Rebate*. Many elderly patients will be at risk of disconnection of gas and/or electricity due to non-payment. In these cases, the patient or their relatives should be advised to contact the energy company straight away, or to get in touch with the local authority when the utility bills are paid as part of a rental agreement. Gas and electricity companies are obliged to give priority service to elderly customers on request.
Home modification	If the occupant requires home modification due to illness, the local authority can be asked for a *Disabled Facilities Grant*.
Transport	Off-peak local bus transport is generally free for those aged 60 and over. Nationally, schemes such as the Senior Citizen's Railcard offer discounted travel.

Table 13.4 UK benefits (*Continued*)

Attendance Allowance	Attendance Allowance is available for people aged 65 and over who need help or supervision with personal care. It can be claimed regardless of whether the person is, at the time, receiving this help or not.
Carer's Allowance	Carer's Allowance is paid to carers for people receiving Attendance Allowance. The claimant must be providing care for over 35 hours a week, and must not earn above a threshold amount. If the carer is already receiving other benefits, these benefits may be increased rather than a specific Carer's Allowance being paid.
Residential and nursing home costs	If a person's savings are above a certain level, they are liable to pay the full costs of residential care. Patients on Section 117 are exempt from this rule.

Same-sex couples

The Civil Partnership Act 2004 came into effect in December 2005. Same-sex couples in a Civil Partnership are now entitled to the same benefit rights as opposite-sex couples.

These issues can be particularly sensitive for an elderly same-sex couple who may in the past have faced criminal proceedings because of their lifestyle. Polari (www.polari.org), an organisation working for better care for older gay men, lesbians, bisexuals and transgendered people, is able to offer support and advice.

Accommodation

Many (but not all) elderly people will need to move into some form of supported accommodation as they grow older. However, it is generally considered to be in the best interests of older people that they are supported in their own home for as long as it is possible and in keeping with their wishes. Help at home may be arranged privately, or provided by the local authority. Paid carers are not able to dispense medication, although they can supervise the patient taking it.

If and when the time comes to move to a more supported environment, several choices are available (Table 13.5). An individual may lack capacity to decide the most appropriate accommodation, and in these situations it is best to consult with relatives wherever possible.

Brief respite admissions for patients with dementia can be of benefit to both patients and carers and are normally arranged by social services, although patients are sometimes admitted to hospital for respite. Elderly servicemen and women may be eligible for respite accommodation in one of the Royal British Legion's care homes or welfare break centres.

Table 13.5 Accommodation choices

Accommodation	Features
Sheltered accommodation	Residents essentially live independently in their own flat. There is usually a resident warden and emergency alarm system and some facilities may be shared. Usually, residents can arrange for external carers if necessary but if the level of care needed is high, residential or nursing home accommodation may be more appropriate.
Residential Home	Supervision and certain services such as meals and laundry provided. Some residential homes have registration to accommodate patients with dementia.
Nursing Home	Registered nurse on site leading team to provide specialist care and supervision for people with chronic medical needs or disability. May have registration to care for people with dementia.

The Elderly Accommodation Counsel (www.eac.org.uk) is a charity that can provide advice to patients and their families regarding accommodation.

Further reading

Age Concern www.ageconcern.co.uk

Casarett D, Kapo J and Kaplan A (2005) Appropriate use of artificial nutrition and hydration – fundamental principles and recommendations *New Engl J Med* 353: 2607–2612.

DVLA Drivers Medical Group *For Medical Practitioners: at a Glance Guide to the Current Medical Standards of Fitness to Drive* Swansea, DVLA www.dvla.gov.uk/media/pdf/medical/aagv1.pdf.

Murray B and Jacoby R (2002) The interface between old age psychiatry and the law *Adv Psychiat Treat* 8: 271–280.

Polari www.polari.org.

Shickle D (2006) The Mental Capacity Act 2005 *Clin Med* 6: 169–173.

The Mental Capacity Act 2005 www.opsi.gov.uk/acts/acts2005/20050009.htm.

The Mental Capacity Act Code of Practice www.justice.gov.uk/guidance/mca-code-of-practice.htm.

The Royal College of Psychiatrists *The Mental Health Team* www.rcpsych.ac.uk/ mentalhealthin-formation/thementalhealthteam.aspx.

UK Government Public Services www.direct.gov.uk.

14

Physical Illness and Old Age Psychiatry

Physical illness and its relationship to psychiatric illness are particularly relevant in old age psychiatry. Many physical conditions may present with psychiatric symptoms, and similarly psychiatric illness can present with physical complaints. Furthermore, psychiatric illness can impact on the course and the outcome of physical illness and vice versa.

This chapter briefly outlines a number of important interactions between physical and psychiatric symptoms and illnesses, covering:

- Delirium

- Vascular disease

- Neurological disease

The Old Age Psychiatry Handbook   Joanne Rodda, Niall Boyce, and Zuzana Walker
© 2008 John Wiley & Sons, Ltd

- Rheumatological disease

- Endocrinological disease

- Nutritional deficiency

- Neoplastic disease

- Palliative care.

Delirium

Delirium (also known as *Acute Confusional State*) is common in the elderly. It is characterised by rapid onset of symptoms (hours/days), with an altered level of consciousness,
global disturbance of cognition, fluctuating course, perceptual abnormalities and evidence of an underlying physical cause. It is often mistaken for dementia or psychiatric
illness and patients with pre-existing dementia are particularly vulnerable in this regard.
As well as caring for a group that is at relatively high risk of delirium, members of the old
age psychiatry team are often asked to assist in the management of patients with delirium on general wards. A clear understanding of the causes, features and management is
therefore essential.

Epidemiology

Estimates of the prevalence of delirium in elderly patients vary depending on setting.
Delirium is relatively rare in the community, with a prevalence of around 1 %, but very
common in hospital where it affects up to one in four of elderly patients. Estimates of
mortality vary from 22–76 %. Up to 50 % of hospital in-patients with delirium will not
have fully recovered at the time of discharge.

Risk factors

Table 14.1 lists the major risk factors for delirium in old age. Older patients are at
greater risk of developing delirium, probably because brain function is compromised by
neurodegeneration.

Causes

There are numerous causes of delirium; common examples are listed in Table 14.2. It
is thought that medication and acute infections are the most frequent causes. Delirium
may be the result of multiple factors, and ideally all of these should be recognised and
addressed in the treatment plan.

Table 14.1 Risk factors for delirium

Patient characteristics	Age over 65
	Male sex
	Functional dependence
	Polypharmacy
Physical illness	Visual and hearing impairment
	Immobility
	Urinary catheter
	Hip fracture/trauma
	Dehydration
	Stroke
	Metabolic abnormalities
	Low postoperative oxygen saturation
	Past history of delirium
Psychiatric illness	Alcoholism or other substance misuse
	Depression
	Dementia

Common examples of *drugs* that may cause delirium are listed in Table 14.3. In some cases, prescribed medicine may cause delirium even when the dose or type of medication has not been changed, because of reduced hepatic or renal clearance secondary to ageing or illness.

Table 14.2 Common causes of delirium

Cause	Examples
Systemic infection	Chest infection, urinary tract infection, cellulitis
Drugs	Prescribed drugs – see Table 14.3
	Intoxication with alcohol and/or prescribed or illicit substances
Cardiovascular	Myocardial infarction
	Cardiac failure
Neurological	Stroke or subsequent complications
	Head trauma, e.g. subdural haematoma
	Raised intracranial pressure/space-occupying lesions
	Epilepsy
	Intracranial infection: meningitis, encephalitis
Metabolic imbalance	Hyponatraemia, hypoglycaemia, anaemia, renal or hepatic insufficiency
Endocrinological	Hypothyroidism, hyperthyroidism, hypopituitarism, hypo/hyperparathyroidism
Substance withdrawal	Alcohol (delirium tremens, page 141 and 253)
	Hypnotics and barbiturates
Other	Hypoxia, dehydration, pain, constipation, acute complications of malignancy, nutritional deficiencies

Table 14.3 Medications associated with delirium

Analgesics	NSAIDs, opiate analgesics (especially pethidine)
Psychotropics	Antidepressants (especially tricyclics), antipsychotics, benzodiazepines, lithium
Cardiovascular medication	Beta blockers, captopril, digoxin, furosemide, isosorbide dinitrate, nifedipine
Respiratory medication	Theophylline
Gastrointestinal medication	Antiemetics (e.g. hyoscine), antidiarrhoeal agents and irritable bowel syndrome treatments containing antimuscarinics, anti-H_2 drugs used for dyspepsia (cimetidine, ranitidine), laxatives
Antiplatelet and anticoagulant drugs	Dipyridamole, warfarin
Steroids	Prednisolone
Antibiotics	Fluoroquinolones
Other	Antiparkinsonian drugs (e.g. L-dopa) Muscle relaxants Older antihistamines (e.g. chlorpheniramine) Ophthalmic medication containing antimuscarinic agents (e.g. atropine) Some herbal over-the-counter medications. Oseltamivir (Tamiflu)

Of note, delirium may also occur as a result of prescribed psychotropic drugs. Where relevant, it is important to exclude *lithium toxicity*, *serotonin syndrome and neuroleptic malignant syndrome* (Chapter 10).

Pathophysiology

Given the heterogeneous causes of delirium, it is unlikely that there is a single pathogenic process common to all cases. There is some evidence that low acetylcholine levels are involved in the process of delirium, and preliminary evidence points to possible benefit from the use of cholinesterase inhibitors in prevention of delirium. Other proposed mechanisms include dopaminergic excess, hypercortisolism, and altered blood brain barrier permeability due to cytokines. There is an association between right-sided brain lesions and delirium.

Clinical features and diagnosis

The onset of delirium is usually rapid (hours/days) and the clinical picture varies widely from patient to patient. It is helpful to think in terms of seven core areas of impairment, these are outlined in Table 14.4.

Table 14.4 Clinical features of delirium

Consciousness	Impaired consciousness, typically fluctuates and often worse in the evening Alertness may be low or high Reduced concentration Disturbance of sleep/wake cycle
Disorientation	Occurs almost without exception Disorientation in time and place is most common, disorientation in person in more severe cases
Thinking	Usually slow and disorganised Fleeting delusions may occur Speech usually ⇓ (may be ⇑) in speed, is often incoherent and rambling
Memory	Impaired, particularly working memory (digit span) and short term memory (of recent events) Mixing of memories and false recall can occur
Behaviour	May be agitation, irritability, wandering and aggression Subdued and hypoactive in some cases Other psychomotor disturbances such as stereotypies may be observed
Perception	Visual distortions, illusions and transient hallucinations Abnormalities in other modalities are less common
Emotion	Varies from apathy to the extremes of euphoria, irritability and outright hostility Low mood, anxiety and emotional lability are common

Delirium can be divided into three subtypes based on the clinical presentation:

• Hypoactive, characterised by lethargy and a marked decrease in motor activity

• Hyperactive, characterised by marked agitation and vigilance

• Mixed.

There is a risk that hypoactive patients may be seen as "non-problematic", so the delirium may not be recognised. Delirium may also escape detection if the patient's behaviour feeds into prejudices about age- or disease-appropriate behaviour. Other patients at risk of being overlooked are those aged 80 or above, those with visual impairment, and patients with dementia.

Important differential diagnoses of delirium include *depression*, *psychosis* and *dementia*. It is also important to rule out non-medical causes of apparently inappropriate behaviour:

• Simple misunderstandings (for example regarding theft, sadly common in hospitals).

• Hearing/visual impairment.

• Culturally appropriate phenomena that do not require treatment (for example, praying or "conversing" pleasantly with dead relatives – see the section on palliative care).

Regardless of the subtype, the principles of management outlined below are the same.

ICD-10 and DSM-IV outline criteria for diagnosis of delirium: these are summarised in Boxes 14.1 and 14.2.

Box 14.1 ICD-10 criteria for delirium

For a diagnosis of delirium, symptoms (mild to severe) should be present in each of the following areas:

1. Impairment of consciousness and attention.

2. Global disturbance of cognition.

3. Psychomotor disturbance.

4. Disturbance of the sleep/wake cycle.

5. Emotional disturbances.

Box 14.2 DSM-IV criteria for delirium

1. Consciousness disturbed.

2. Change in cognition or perceptual disturbance not accounted for by dementia.

3. Development of illness over short period of time (hours to days) and fluctuating course.

4. History, physical examination, or laboratory findings support general medical condition, substance intoxication/withdrawal, or multiple aetiologies.

5. If there is insufficient evidence for any of the categories listed in (4), or if the cause is not listed in (4) (e.g. delirium secondary to sensory deprivation) a diagnosis of "delirium not otherwise specified" is given.

The use of rating scales can also be helpful in the diagnosis of delirium. The MMSE is widely used, but more specific assessment tools include the *Confusion Assessment Method* (CAM), the *Organic Brain Syndrome Scale*, and the *Delirium Rating Scale*. The CAM is a fast and easy-to-use scale, and is given in full in Box 14.3.

Box 14.3   The Confusion Assessment Method (CAM)

Delirium is diagnosed if the patient has:

1. Acute onset and fluctuating course
and

2. Inattention
and

3. Disorganised thinking OR altered level of consciousness.

Other delirium symptoms:
disorientation, memory impairment, perceptual disturbances, psychomotor agitation or retardation, altered sleep/wake cycle.

History

When delirium is suspected, it is important to identify and characterise the clinical features outlined above with the emphasis on:

- The nature of *onset* and *course* of problems

- Any *diurnal variation* of symptoms

- The level of functioning prior to onset of delirium

- A full *past medical and psychiatric history*, including any past episodes of delirium

- A full *drug history* including any recent changes to medication

- *Alcohol* history to exclude intoxication or withdrawal (see delirium tremens, below).

This information may not be available from the patient, and a collateral history from nursing staff and/or relatives as well as a thorough review of any available medical notes is essential.

Examination and investigations

A great deal of information regarding the cause of delirium may be gained from the history as outlined above. Further assessment includes:

- Full physical examination.

- Infection screen (blood, urine and stool cultures and chest x-ray).

- Other blood tests: full blood count, glucose, renal and liver function tests, inflammatory markers, thyroid function test, calcium and phosphate.

- PR examination and abdominal x-ray if severe constipation suspected.

- Use of assessment scales (e.g. MMSE, CAM – see above).

Other investigations (e.g. neuroimaging) will be guided by the clinical picture.

Management

For patients in the community or on a psychiatric ward, admission or transfer to a medical ward is often necessary. In many cases the psychiatric team is asked to assist in the management of patients on a general medical or surgical ward. It is almost always better for the patient to remain on that ward rather than to be transferred to a psychiatric unit. In this situation, the role of the physician is to treat the *underlying causes* of the delirium, and the role of the psychiatrist is to offer advice on *supportive care* and *emergency symptom control*.

If the patient lacks *capacity to consent*, treatment should be given under the Mental Capacity Act 2005 (in the past, common law was used, see page 230). Use of the Mental Health Act is not appropriate.

There are three key areas of focus in the management of delirium, and these are outlined in more detail below:

1. Look for and treat the underlying cause(s).

2. Non-pharmacological interventions.

3. Pharmacological interventions.

1. Look for and treat underlying causes

Ultimately, the underlying cause needs to be identified and treated before symptoms will resolve. Medication is reviewed and minimised. Pain management, hydration and oxygenation are optimised whilst the ongoing assessment aims to identify any other cause of the delirium.

2. Non-pharmacological management of symptoms of delirium

There are a number of practical steps that are considered by general consensus to be good practice in the management of delirium, shown in Box 14.4.

Box 14.4   Good practice in management of delirium

Nurse the patient closely, 1:1 if necessary, in a quiet side-room with consistent reassurance and reorientation. Aim for consistency of care staff to minimise confusion.

Have familiar objects from the patient's home in the room. Involve family and friends to promote security/orientation.

Make sure the patient has glasses/hearing aids where necessary.

If possible, mobilise to avoid consequences of immobility, e.g. deep vein thrombosis, chest infection, and pressure sores.

---

3. Pharmacological management of symptoms of delirium

The decision to use pharmacological management strategies should be taken on a balance of risk to the patient from the medication versus the risk of harm as a result of continuing problematic or dangerous behaviour. Whenever drugs are used, it is essential to monitor regularly for side effects and any improvement in symptoms. If symptoms do not respond, the drug should be stopped.

Antipsychotic drugs (page 186)   Antipsychotic drugs are probably the drug of choice for severe agitation and/or aggression in delirium and there is a limited evidence base to support their use. It is important to perform an ECG (where possible) before and during treatment, to identify any QT prolongation or arrhythmia.

Haloperidol is the most commonly used antipsychotic drug in delirium:

- It has the advantage of fewer anticholinergic side effects, minimal cardiovascular side effects, short half-life and no active metabolites.

- There is RCT evidence to support its use in delirium.

- It can be given orally or i.m.

- The starting dose should be low – titrate gradually up from 0.5 mg/day to a maximum of 10 mg/day. If giving as an i.m. injection, halve the dose.

- Assess daily for symptoms of delirium, level of sedation and extrapyramidal side effects (EPSE). Reduce the dose or stop rather than give anticholinergic drugs for EPSE (anticholinergic drugs can induce delirium).

Whilst atypical antipsychotic drugs are less sedating and have fewer EPSE than haloperidol, some have a greater anticholinergic effect, and there are concerns about their safety. Atypicals have been shown to be associated with a higher mortality rate in dementia (compared to placebo) and there is little evidence to support their use in delirium over haloperidol. When prescribed, the starting dose for risperidone is 0.5–1 mg o.d. and for quetiapine, 25 mg.

Benzodiazepines (page 193)   Benzodiazepines may be helpful in the management of delirium, although haloperidol is usually more appropriate for more severely disturbed patients. They are also used in the management of delirium related to alcohol/sedative drugs withdrawal, and are the drug of choice in patients for whom antipsychotics are contraindicated (e.g. due to EPSE, hepatic insufficiency).

The use of benzodiazepines is somewhat controversial, as side effects may exacerbate confusion and disorientation and result in falls or worsening of respiratory failure. Tolerance and dependence are less of an issue in the short term.

If benzodiazepines are used, start with a short-acting drug at a low dose, for example 0.5 mg lorazepam, maximum dose b.d. Give orally where possible and make sure the ward has flumazenil in stock, particularly if using the intramuscular route. Patients must be monitored carefully for signs of respiratory depression or worsening confusion and disorientation.

Outcome

Delirium is associated with several adverse outcomes, shown in Box 14.5.

Box 14.5   Adverse outcomes associated with delirium

Prolonged hospitalisation.

Poor recovery post-surgery.

Increased likelihood of discharge to an institution.

Increased morbidity/mortality.

There are many factors that contribute to the mortality associated with delirium (Box 14.6):

> **Box 14.6 Factors contributing to mortality in delirium**
>
> The patient's delirious symptoms can make diagnosis and treatment of the underlying medical condition difficult.
>
> Wandering and agitation may lead to falls.
>
> In hypoactive forms of delirium, inactivity may lead to chest infections, bedsores and deep vein thrombosis.
>
> Delirium in old age has been associated with increased risk of developing dementia (this may be related to the concept of cognitive reserve, page 37).

Cessation of the more dramatic symptoms of delirium is not synonymous with recovery. Elderly patients who have had delirium may need continued rehabilitation after discharge and future medical treatment should address the risk factors for further episodes of delirium.

Delirium Tremens

Delirium tremens (Box 14.7) is a potentially fatal complication of alcohol withdrawal. It generally develops one to seven days (peak 48 hours) after alcohol intake is dramatically reduced or stopped by a heavy user. Hospital admission is a frequent cause of imposed abstinence.

Vascular disease

Cardiovascular disease

One quarter of patients who have had a myocardial infarction (MI) or who are undergoing angiography have minor depression, whilst another quarter have major depression. Heart failure and hypertension have also been associated with depression in some studies.

Some research suggests that depression may be a risk factor for as well as an adverse effect of cardiac disease. For management of depression, see Chapter 3. Important cautions and contraindications of antidepressants are summarised in Chapter 10.

Patients with myocardial infarction or hypoxia resulting from poorly controlled heart failure may present with delirium.

Box 14.7   Delirium tremens (DTs, see also page 141)

Prevalence

DTs occur in 5 % of cases of alcohol withdrawal.

Reported mortality is 5–15 %.

Pathophysiology

Sudden alcohol cessation removes the inhibitory effect of alcohol (via GABA and NMDA receptors) on the central nervous system. The increase in excitatory neural activity is thought to lead to the symptoms of DTs.

Presentation

Prodromal symptoms are anxiety, tremor and sweating. These are followed by fever, clouding of consciousness, tachycardia, persistent visual, tactile and auditory hallucinations and, in some cases, paranoid delusions. There may be associated metabolic disturbances and fits. Be aware that 50 % of patients with delirium tremens have an associated trauma or infection.

Treatment

The patient should be managed on a medical ward or ITU.

A gradually reducing dose of a benzodiazepine such as chlordiazepoxide at a dose titrated to symptoms within recommended limits is the first line of treatment. For patients with marked hepatic impairment a shorter-acting benzodiazepine such as oxazepam is appropriate.

Haloperidol can be used cautiously as an additional agent to control psychiatric symptoms such as hallucinations, anxiety and paranoia (however, it reduces seizures threshold).

The patient should also receive supportive care and intravenous B-complex vitamins (Pabrinex).

Stroke

Stroke causes a rapidly developing focal impairment of CNS function. If the impairment resolves within 24 hours, the event is classified as a Transient Ischaemic Attack (TIA).

Incidence

Stroke is common, with an incidence of 2 in 1000 annually.

Aetiology

The majority of strokes (90 %) are due to infarction. The remainder are haemorrhagic.

Risk factors

Risk factors for stroke include:

- Hypertension

- Structural cardiac disease (e.g. recent MI)

- Hyperlipidaemia

- Smoking

- Old age

- High alcohol intake

- Diabetes mellitus

- Anticoagulant therapy (haemorrhagic stroke *only*)

- Family history.

Presentation

Acute   The manifestations of stroke include:

- Weakness or paralysis

- Ataxia

- Speech disorders (dysphasia, dysarthria)

- Impaired swallow (dysphagia)

- Visual impairment

- Sensory impairment

- Reduced level of consciousness

Table 14.5   Effects of cerebral artery occlusion

Vessel occluded	Effects
Anterior cerebral artery	Contralateral hemiparesis, leg > arm Cortical sensory loss Motor dysphasia Frontal lobe dysfunction
Middle cerebral artery	Contralateral hemiparesis, arm > leg Contralateral hemianaesthesia Contralateral hemianopia Dysphasia (dominant hemisphere)
Posterior cerebral artery	Contralateral hemianopia, visual perseveration (palinopsia), agnosias, spatial disorientation, memory impairment

Patients with these features will normally present initially to the medical team. However, in some patients, stroke may present initially with abrupt cognitive and behavioural changes.

The effects of occlusion of the anterior, middle and cerebral arteries are given in Table 14.5.

Following stroke patients frequently develop psychiatric complications.

Box 14.8   Complications of stroke

Depression/anxiety

Emotional lability

Apathy

Behavioural disturbance

Personality changes

Cognitive impairment

Post-stroke depression is discussed on page 63, whilst the effect of cerebrovascular disease on cognition and personality is summarised in Chapter 2.

Table 14.6 Clinical effects of lesions to specific lobes

Site of lesion	Manifestation
Frontal lobe	Personality or behavioural change. Grasp reflex/Broca's expressive aphasia/forced utilisation. Contralateral weakness/paresis if primary motor cortex affected.
Parietal lobe	Either lobe: visuospatial agnosia, contralateral cortical sensory loss, dysgraphaesthesia. Dominant: dysphasia, apraxia, finger agnosia, dyscalculia, R-L disorientation, agraphia. Non-dominant: anosognosia, contralateral neglect, prosopagnosia, dressing dyspraxia.
Temporal lobe	Upper homonymous visual fields defects. Auditory/vestibular loss in superior/marginal gyrus. Dysphasia. Impairment of prosody. Memory impairment: −verbal (dominant temporal lobe) −visual (non-dominant temporal lobe).
Cerebellum	Ataxia, intention tremor. Cerebellar cognitive affective syndrome (impaired executive function, spatial cognition, blunted affect, aggramatism/dysprosodia).

Important effects of damage to the different lobes of the brain are summarised in Table 14.6. Details of basic tests of lobe function are given in Appendix 2, page 285.

Treatment

Acute   It has been clearly shown that stroke patients managed on specialist stroke units have a better outcome than those managed on general medical or geriatric wards.

Treatment of acute ischaemic stroke is becoming more active with the advent of thrombolysis for mild to moderately severe cases. Furthermore, for "malignant" middle cerebral artery territory infarction, surgical decompression of the affected hemisphere has been shown to be beneficial.

Chronic   The primary aims of post-stroke medical treatment are rehabilitation and secondary prevention.

As a psychiatrist, it is possible to assist in optimising function through the recognition and treatment of depression and anxiety (see Chapter 3). The role of anticholinesterase medication in vascular dementia is still unclear (see page 46).

Box 14.9   Secondary prevention of stroke

Patients with ischaemic stroke should receive antiplatelet medication (e.g. aspirin, clopidogrel, dipyridamole). Anticoagulant therapy (warfarin) is indicated in specific cases (principally atrial fibrillation).

Hypertension and hypercholesterolaemia should be treated. It has also been shown that normotensive individuals with normal cholesterol levels benefit from anti-hypertensive and statin therapy.

Patients should also be advised regarding dietary changes and smoking cessation.

Chronic subdural haematoma

A *subdural haematoma (SDH)* is caused by bleeding from the bridging veins between the dura and arachnoid mater. Elderly people are at particular risk of chronic subdural haematoma, even after a relatively minor head injury. Other risk factors include chronic alcoholism and coagulopathies or anticoagulant treatment.

Chronic subdural haematoma can lead to a clinical picture similar to delirium or dementia, with progressive and/or fluctuating cognitive deficits and drowsiness. Onset is usually insidious. There may be associated headache and neurological signs (for example, ataxia, extensor plantar reflex). Surgical intervention (evacuation of haematoma) may be warranted.

Neurological disease

Epilepsy

Old age psychiatrists frequently encounter patients with "funny turns". The aetiology is not always clear and may include epilepsy, syncope, falls, vertigo, silent MIs and TIAs. A diagnosis of epilepsy is therefore frequently missed.

From the age of 55, prevalence of epilepsy increases such that prevalence at age 85 and over (1.2–2 %) is twice that of the general population. It has also been estimated that 8 % of nursing home residents experience seizures.

In patients with *known epilepsy*, new psychiatric symptoms of dementia, depression or psychosis may be independent or secondary to epilepsy.

The most common causes of *new onset epilepsy* in elderly patients are given in Box 14.10.

Box 14.10 Common causes of new onset epilepsy in the elderly

Cerebrovascular disease (25–30 %)

Metabolic derangement

Brain tumours

Head trauma

Dementia

Medications (including antidepressants and antipsychotics)

CNS infection

Clinical features

As the majority of new-onset seizures in the elderly result from focal pathology, onset tends to be partial. Secondary generalisation may follow. Epileptic symptoms in the elderly may therefore be mistaken for psychiatric disorders.

Common presenting symptoms include those shown in Box 14.11.

Box 14.11 Common symptoms of new onset epilepsy in the elderly

Acute behavioural changes (may be subtle)

Confusion

Mental slowing

Memory disturbance

Faints

Investigations

- Routine blood tests and ECG should be undertaken in all patients.

- MRI brain (CT is not a suitable investigation).

- EEG is not a routine requirement as it is often unremarkable and rarely contributes to making a diagnosis of epilepsy. Video EEG telemetry may be indicated in difficult cases.

Treatment

Medication review is necessary as seizures may be a side effect of several medications including antidepressants and antipsychotics.

Suspected cases should be referred to a neurologist for an opinion on the diagnosis and advice about the appropriate anticonvulsant treatment.

Differential diagnoses

Physical illnesses whose presentation may resemble epilepsy include those shown in Table 14.7.

Old age psychiatrists may be asked to treat patients with psychogenic disorders, although they occur comparatively rarely in old age: (Table 14.8)

Table 14.7　Conditions with presentation resembling epilepsy

Cause	Notes
Vascular	Stroke/TIA Vasovagal syncope Orthostatic hypotension Arrhythmias Structural disease (e.g. aortic stenosis)
Neurological	Migraine Narcolepsy Restless legs and periodic limb movements of sleep Transient global amnesia
Sleep disorders	Obstructive sleep apnoea Hypnic jerks REM sleep disorders

Table 14.8　Psychogenic disorders that may be confused with epilepsy

Cause	Notes
Psychogenic amnesia	Involves unusual, selective patterns of autobiographical memory loss
Psychogenic non-epileptic attacks (PNEA)	Non-epileptic seizures difficult to distinguish from true epilepsy

Table 14.9 Core clinical features of Parkinson's disease

Akinesia	Observable poverty or lack of movement. Includes reduced movements of facial expression (hypomimia)
Bradykinesia	Slowness of movement, which can be observed and tested formally
Rigidity	A symptom (stiffness) and a sign, which can affect the limbs, neck and trunk. In Parkinson's disease, limbs will be affected usually asymmetrically. "Cogwheeling" rigidity may be regarded as the modification of rigidity by tremor
Tremor	Classically a rest tremor (4–6 Hz), which abates initially when the limb is moved to adopt a posture or carry out an action. Visually asymmetrical
Postural abnormalities	Most commonly a stooped posture (but there are many differential diagnoses of this sign)
Impaired postural control	Commonly includes difficulty getting in and out of seats, and leads to falls
Abnormalities of gait	Difficulty initiating walking, small paces initially, impaired arm swing, and increased number of paces required to turn around

Other consequences of akinesia, bradykinesia and rigidity include micrographia, dysphonia, dysarthria and dribbling

Parkinson's disease and related conditions

Dementia with Lewy bodies (DLB), Parkinson's disease with dementia (PDD) and Parkinson's disease form part of a spectrum of Lewy body disorders. DLB and PDD are discussed on page 46. The physical presentation of Parkinson's disease is summarised below.

Presentation

The core clinical features of Parkinson's disease are:

Common psychiatric symptoms of Parkinson's disease include those given in Table 14.10.

Other non-motor symptoms of Parkinson's disease include those shown in Box 14.12.

Incidence/prevalence

Annual incidence of idiopathic Parkinson's disease is 20 in 100 000. The majority of these cases will be individuals in their mid 50s or above. Prevalence in the over 60s is 1–2 %.

Table 14.10 Common psychiatric symptoms of Parkinson's disease

Parkinson's disease	Dementia of Parkinson's disease	Medication side effects
Apathy/lack of initiative (abulia) Depression/anxiety/panic attacks (10–45 %) Slowing of thinking (bradyphrenia)		
	Hallucinations/delusions/illusions (40 %) Delirium Disinhibited behaviour Cognitive impairment	
	Obsessional features Change in personality	

Box 14.12   Other non-motor symptoms of Parkinson's disease

Sleep disorders (REM sleep Behaviour Disorder, excessive daytime sleepiness)

Associated autonomic failure (postural hypotension, sexual dysfunction, failure of bladder control)

Sensory symptoms

Aetiology

Parkinson's disease is a progressive, idiopathic neurodegenerative disorder, the molecular pathology of which includes accumulation of dysnuclein in affected neurones. The dopaminergic nigrostriatal neurones in the substantia nigra are particularly affected.

The core features of Parkinson's disease (also referred to as Parkinsonism, see Table 14.9) can also be present in a number of other conditions (see Box 14.13). Parkinsonian side effects of antipsychotics, antiemetics and other medications are very common and should always be considered in the differential diagnosis of Parkinson's disease.

Treatment

The main drugs used for Parkinson's disease are listed in Table 14.11.

> ## Box 14.13 Conditions causing Parkinsonism
>
> Idiopathic Parkinson's disease
>
> Drug induced Parkinsonism
>
> Vascular Parkinsonism
>
> Progressive supranuclear palsy
>
> Multisystem atrophy
>
> Corticobasal degeneration
>
> Normal pressure hydrocephalus
>
> Traumatic encephalopathy (repeated head injury)
>
> Sequela of hypoxia/carbon monoxide poisoning

Table 14.11 Side effects of medication used in Parkinson's disease

Medication	Side effects
Levodopa (L-DOPA) (Usually given with a dopa–decarboxylase inhibitor to reduce peripheral L-DOPA-to-dopamine conversion)	Motor fluctuations/dyskinesia Psychiatric side effects (see below) Other: nausea/vomiting (usually transient), postural hypotension, exacerbation of peptic ulcers, sweating, and dark urine/sweat
Dopamine agonists (Pergolide, cabergoline, ropinorole, pramipexole, rotigotine)	Psychiatric side effects Postural hypotension Vasospasm, ankle swelling, pleuropulmonary/retroperitoneal fibrosis (rare)
Monoamine oxidase B inhibitors (Selegeline)	Increase in L-DOPA side effects
Catechol-O methytransferase (COMT) inhibitors (entacapone, tolcapone)	Increase in L-DOPA side effects Nausea/vomiting Hepatic toxicity with tolcapone
Amantadine	Psychiatric side effects (especially nervousness, inability to concentrate, confusion/hallucinations) Convulsions Nausea/GI disturbance
Anticholinergics (benzhexol, orphenadrine)	Psychiatric side effects (especially delirium) Dyskinesia, mydriasis (contraindicated in narrow angle glaucoma), dry mouth, constipation *Generally not used in elderly patients (page 246)*

Psychiatric side effects of antiparkinsonian medication include:

Box 14.14   Psychiatric side effects of antiparkinsonian medication

Vivid dreams/nightmares

Illusions and visual hallucinations

Delusions

Mood disorders including depression, anxiety and hypomania/mania

Schizophreniform psychosis

Increased libido

Increased tendency towards gambling

If it is suspected that psychiatric symptoms are due to antiparkinsonian medication, it is best to contact the patient's neurologist to discuss the risks and benefits of reducing medication. In practice, the balance between ameliorating motor symptoms and worsening psychiatric symptoms can be difficult to achieve.

Normal pressure hydrocephalus (NPH)

Normal pressure hydrocephalus is a potentially treatable cause of impaired cognitive and motor function.

Aetiology

NPH involves the slow, chronic dilatation of brain ventricles due to intermittent small increases of CSF pressure. CSF pressure measured by standard manometry at lumbar puncture is normal. In most cases NPH is idiopathic, but it can be a late sequela of trauma, meningitis or haemorrhage.

Presentation

Patients with NPH classically present with a progressive pattern of:

> **Box 14.15 Clinical features of normal pressure hydrocephalus**
>
> Dementia
>
> Gait ataxia
>
> Urinary incontinence
>
> Extensor plantar reflexes

Investigations

Head MRI shows ventricular enlargement. The diagnosis is often extremely difficult to make on imaging grounds as:

- Ventricular dilatation is also seen in atrophy.

- Atrophy and NPH may co-exist.

- In NPH there may be "external" hydrocephalus with enlargement of the Sylvian fissures and some cortical sulci (which looks indistinguishable from atrophy).

Treatment

The dementia and ataxia secondary to NPH is *potentially reversible* with ventriculo-peritoneal shunting. However this procedure carries a high risk of complications, and is not suitable for all patients.

CNS Infection

Although comparatively rare, there are several important infective causes of neuropsychiatric presentation in the elderly.

Table 14.12 Clinical progression of syphilis

Primary – incubation period three weeks	Chance (painless ulcer) at site of infection resolves spontaneously.
Secondary – six to eight weeks later	Generalised maculopapular rash, generalised lymphadenopathy, condylomata lata (infectious plaques), fever, arthralgias, weight loss.
Latent syphilis	Patient asymptomatic, but still has positive serology.
Tertiary syphilis (five to twenty years)	Gummata (focal hard nodular lesions) in liver, skin, bone, spleen), aortitis, neurosyphilis (see below).

Neurosyphilis

Neurosyphilis is caused by Treponema pallidum. Although effective prevention and treatment methods are available, the effect of syphilis on the central nervous system (neurosyphilis) may still present to psychiatry.

Incidence   Syphilis is comparatively rare in the UK with diagnosis rates of around 1 per 100 000.

Presentation   The classical pattern of progression for syphilis is given in Table 14.12.
  An old age psychiatrist is most likely to see a patient with neurosyphilis. Symptoms include:

- *Psychiatric:* general paresis (grandiosity, cognitive impairment), dementia, manic psychosis with mood-congruent delusions.

- *Neurological:* headache, cranial neuropathy, stroke, seizures, myelopathy, radiculopathy, dorsal root ganglionitis (tabes dorsalis – sensory ataxia, areflexia, impaired pain sensation).

- *Ocular:* abnormalities including (in 26 %) the Argyll Roberston pupil, which is small, irregular, and unreactive to light but accommodates.

Diagnosis   Syphilis is diagnosed serologically through the Venereal Disease Research Laboratory test (VDRL) or rapid plasma regain (RPR) tests. Diagnosis is subsequently confirmed by fluorescent treponemal antibody absorption (FTA-ABS) or microhaemagglutination assay (MHA-TP). If neurosyphilis is suspected, the VDRL can be used to test cerebrospinal fluid.

Treatment   Treatment should be given in liaison with local sexual health specialists. It generally comprises penicillin G given with prednisolone, and screening of the patient's sexual partner(s) and children.

HIV

Whilst HIV management has not formed a major part of geriatric medicine and psychiatry in the past, current evidence suggests that it will be one of the challenges of the future. Patients with HIV may present with a variety of psychiatric symptoms, including HIV-associated dementia (HAD), minor cognitive-motor disorder (MCMD), HIV psychosis and depression.

Treatment

Dementia   Although HIV-related dementia does respond to highly active antiretroviral therapy (HAART), HAART does not protect fully against the development of HAD or MCMD. It has been suggested that cholinesterase inhibitors and memantine may be of use in HAD, but as yet no RCT evidence is available.

Psychosis   Whether psychosis in HIV patients is directly related to HIV pathology or not, antipsychotic treatment is generally appropriate. However, patients with HIV are particularly sensitive to extrapyramidal side effects, and this problem appears to be especially pronounced in older patients. It is therefore recommended that low-dose atypical antipsychotics should be the first line of treatment.

Other infections

TB, Herpes simplex virus (HSV 1), Epstein-Barr virus, measles, influenza and prion disease may also cause rapidly progressing psychiatric illness in the elderly.

Rheumatological disease

Rheumatological illness itself or drugs used to treat it may result in a psychiatric presentation. Alternatively, advice regarding management of psychiatric symptoms in rheumatological illness may be sought by medical colleagues.

Temporal arteritis

Temporal arteritis (giant cell arteritis) is a necrotising vasculitis common in the over 55s in Northern Europe, where it has a prevalence of 17–18 per 100 000. It mostly occurs in white people.

Presentation

The most common presenting feature is headache, which is initially quite severe. It can affect any part of the head, often the temples or the back of the head. The headache may be accompanied by scalp tenderness, and sometimes jaw claudication. Systemic symptoms include malaise, aches and pains in muscles and joints, cough, weight loss and fever.

Headache, malaise, and weight loss are also common psychiatric symptoms, and it is therefore advisable to bear this diagnosis in mind as an important differential in older patients. Presentation of temporal arteritis with psychotic symptoms has been reported.

The serious complications of temporal arteritis are ischaemic optic neuropathy and stroke.

Management

- If temporal arteritis is suspected, request inflammatory markers. Raised ESR and CRP increase the probability of the diagnosis.

- Consult rheumatology colleagues and arrange temporal artery biopsy.

- Usual management is oral prednisolone 40–60 mg/day, reduced depending on patient response one week later.

Systemic lupus erythematosus (SLE)

In contrast with temporal arteritis, SLE becomes less common after the age of 50. However, as neuropsychiatric symptoms are common in SLE patients, it is a differential diagnosis worth bearing in mind for cases of late-onset psychosis.

Prevalence

- SLE has a prevalence of approximately 28 per 100 000, but may be as high as 206/100 000 in Afro-Caribbean women.

- Onset usually occurs between the late teens and early 40s.

- The female:male ratio is approximately 9:1. However in older patients there is evidence that this ratio may be reduced.

Presentation

Symptoms of SLE that can present to psychiatry include malaise, headaches, cognitive dysfunction and psychosis. Common clinical features of SLE are given in Table 14.13.

Table 14.13 Common clinical features of SLE

Neuropsychiatric	Psychosis, severe depression, general malaise, headache, seizures, visual disturbance, aseptic meningitis, delirium, coma, dementia.
Neurological	Stroke, myelitis, polyneuropathy.
Dermatological	Malar butterfly rash, photosensitivity, discoid rash, oral/nasal ulcers.
Musculoskeletal	Arthralgia, malaise, myositis, polyarthritis.
Renal	Renal impairment, proteinuria/casts detected.
Cardiopulmonary	Pleuritis, pericarditis.
Haematological	Haemolytic anaemia, leucopaenia, lymphopaenia, thrombocytopaenia.

Investigation

Bloods: FBC usually shows anaemia. ESR and CRP are raised, antinuclear antibodies are positive in 98 %, rheumatoid factor is positive in 30–50 % and DNA binding antibodies are specific for SLE but are present in only 50 % of cases.
Imaging: MRI of brain may show high-signal changes suggestive of vasculopathy.

Management

Management in liaison with medical colleagues involves immunosuppressive medication, and, in the case of psychotic presentation, antipsychotics.

Endocrinological disease

Diabetes mellitus (DM)

There are many ways in which diabetes may be relevant in psychiatry. For example, diabetes can present with mood or behavioural disturbances and there is an association between depression and diabetes (page 63). Patients taking atypical antipsychotics are at increased risk of obesity and type II diabetes. It is therefore important to have some knowledge of its aetiology, symptoms and management in old age psychiatry.

Diabetes mellitus type I

Type I DM usually has onset in children or young adults, is the result of insulin deficiency and is managed by subcutaneous injection of insulin. The long-term complications are similar to type II diabetes. Diabetic ketoacidosis (DKA) is an emergency occurring in type I DM, presenting with hyperglycaemia and gross metabolic disturbances.

Diabetes mellitus type II

Type II diabetes is discussed in more detail in this section as onset is more common in middle and older age and it is a more commonly encountered problem in old age psychiatry than type I diabetes.

Aetiology   DM type II is a multifactorial process leading to gradually increasing insensitivity to insulin. There is a strong genetic component.

Prevalence   The vast majority of cases of DM type II are of adult onset, and prevalence increases with age. In the UK, prevalence is 2 % and rising. It is increased in certain ethnic groups (e.g. Asians).

Risk factors   Risk factors for DM type II include obesity, lack of exercise, genetic factors and certain drugs, e.g. antipsychotics (page 190). The prevalence of DM in patients with schizophrenia or bipolar illness is 2–4 times higher than in the general population. This is most likely the result of environmental factors, lifestyle and genetic predisposition.

Presentation   The majority of patients are over the age of 50 at presentation. The classic triad is of thirst, polyuria and weight loss. However, in type II DM onset is likely to be insidious and the presenting features are often a result of complications of the diabetes, for example visual impairment, neuropathy, staphylococcal skin infections or foot ulcers. Patients may present to a psychiatrist with fatigue and/or low mood, or more acutely with behavioural disturbances secondary to hyperglycaemia.

A hyperosmolar non-ketoacidotic (HONK) state may occur in type II diabetes, sometimes as a presenting feature. It is a metabolic emergency with uncontrolled hyperglycaemia in the absence of ketosis. It may present with mental state changes or even delirium.

Diagnosis   A fasting blood glucose should be taken.

- Below 6 mmol/L – Normal

- 6–7 mmol/L – Impaired glucose tolerance

- 7 mmol/L or above – Diabetes.

In "borderline" cases, it may be necessary to request a glucose tolerance test. A further test is HbA1c, which gives a measure of glucose control over the preceding weeks. A level greater than 7 % is strongly suggestive of diabetes.

Other blood tests are directed at identifying complications and potential exacerbating factors.

Treatment   Management should be discussed with the patient's GP or local diabetes team who will ideally initiate and monitor treatment. Their role will include screening for the presence of complications (below) and providing support and advice to the patient and their family. Medication, especially atypical antipsychotics, should be reviewed.

Essentially, treatment options for glycaemic control are:

- Lifestyle interventions: dietary advice, weight loss, physical activity

- Oral hypoglycaemics, e.g. metformin

- Subcutaneous insulin.

Successful glycaemic control is often a result of a combination of lifestyle changes and oral medication. Patients with type II DM who require insulin have not developed type I DM.

Other important aspects of management are:

- Optimisation of any modifiable vascular risk factors

  - control of hypertension and hypercholesterolaemia

  - smoking cessation.

- Early detection and management of complications.

Complications   DM type II has many complications. These include:

- Macrovascular complications: stroke, ischaemic heart disease, peripheral vascular disease

- Retinopathy

- Nephropathy

- Neuropathy

- Cataracts

- Infections

- Diabetic foot (multifactorial aetiology).

Hypothyroidism

Hypothyroidism (thyroid hormone deficiency) may cause or exacerbate depressive illness or apparent cognitive impairment in the elderly. Its insidious onset may lead to difficulty in diagnosis.

Prevalence

Hypothyroidism is common in the over 60s, with a prevalence of 2–7 %.

Aetiology

The vast majority of cases of hypothyroidism are primary (i.e. due to insufficient thyroid hormone production).

Low circulating levels of thyroid stimulating hormone (TSH) or thyroid releasing hormone (TRH) cause secondary hypothyroidism.

Common causes of hypothyroidism are given in Table 14.14. Of note in old age psychiatry is the role played by *lithium* in drug-induced primary hypothyroidism.

Presentation

Presenting features of hypothyroidism in the elderly are listed in Table 14.15. In all new cases of depression, psychosis and cognitive impairment in the elderly it is important to look for signs of hypothyroidism on the physical examination and to test thyroid function.

Investigation

Thyroid function tests will reveal low T4 and high TSH levels in cases of primary hypothyroidism, whereas with secondary hypothyroidism the low T4 will be accompanied by a low or normal TSH.

Table 14.14 Common causes of hypothyroidism

Primary hypothyroidism	**Acquired**	Autoimmune (Hashimoto's, atrophic, rarely Riedel's)
		Iatrogenic (surgery, radioiodine, carbimazole)
		Iodine deficiency/excess
		Drugs (e.g. lithium)
	Congenital	Thyroid dysgenesis
		Iodine deficiency
		Genetic deficiencies in hormone synthesis
Secondary hypothyroidism	**Hypothalamic disease**	TRH deficiency
	Pituitary disease	TSH deficiency

Table 14.15 Presenting features of hypothyroidism

Psychiatric	Lethargy, mental slowing, depression, cognitive impairment, psychosis ("Myxoedema madness")
Physical	*General* – cold intolerance, weight gain, facial puffiness, husky voice, thinning hair, dry skin *Musculoskeletal* – cramps *Cardiac* – pericardial effusion *Gastrointestinal* – constipation *Neurological* – ataxia, paraesthesia, slow relaxing reflexes, bilateral carpal tunnel syndrome

Management

Patients with hypothyroidism can normally be managed in primary care. Oral thyroxine should be started at a low dose (e.g. 25 micrograms/day) and titrated according to further thyroid function tests and repeated clinical examination.

Hyperthyroidism

Hyperthyroidism is caused by an excess of free thyroid hormones.

Prevalence

Hyperthyroidism has a prevalence of 0.2–2 % in the elderly.

Aetiology

The most common causes of hyperthyroidism in the elderly are toxic uninodular or multinodular goitre and Graves' disease.

Other causes include Hashimoto's thyroiditis and viral thyroiditis. Iatrogenic hyperthyroidism may occur following excess thyroid replacement therapy.

Presentation

The important presenting features of hyperthyroidism are listed in Table 14.16.

Management

- Medication – carbimazole is the first line of treatment in all patients (starting dose usually 40–60 mg/day, titrated according to response). Patients on carbimazole should

Table 14.16 Presenting features of hyperthyroidism

Psychiatric	Anxiety, irritability
Physical	*General* – weight loss, heat intolerance, increased sweating, clubbing, fine tremor, goitre with or without bruit, pretibial myxoedema *Thyroid eye disease* – proptosis, exophthalmos, ophthalmoplegia, visual impairment, corneal ulceration *Cardiovascular* – arrhythmia, cardiomyopathy, heart failure *Gastrointestinal* – diarrhoea *Musculoskeletal* – proximal myopathy

be advised of the 0.1 % risk of agranulocytosis, and that medical advice should be sought *immediately* if sore throat or fever develops.

- Surgery – thyroidectomy.

- Radioiodine.

Cushing's syndrome

Cushing's syndrome results from long-term excessive glucocorticoid exposure.

In elderly patients, the majority of cases of Cushing's syndrome are iatrogenic, although rarely it may be due to endogenous hypersecretion of glucocorticoids. The female:male ratio is 4:1.

Presentation

Table 14.17 Clinical presentation of Cushing's syndrome

Psychiatric	Depression, psychosis, fatigue
Physical	*General* – polydipsia/polyuria *Appearance* – weight gain (centripetal), purple striae, supraclavicular fat pad, thinned hair, moon face, acne, hirsutism, frontal balding, thin skin, easy bruising *Cardiovascular* – hypertension, ischaemic heart disease *Musculoskeletal* – proximal myopathy, evidence of fractures

Diagnosis

Serum electrolyte levels may show hypokalaemia. Blood glucose may be raised. A 24-hour urine collection will reveal a raised level of free cortisol.

Treatment

In iatrogenic cases, discontinuation or reduction of steroids is normally sufficient for treatment. If the excess glucocorticoid secretion is endogenous, it is possible that a pituitary adenoma is present, and specialist endocrinological and surgical management is necessary.

Nutritional deficit

Thiamine deficiency

Elderly patients with and without a history of alcohol misuse are at risk of thiamine deficiency.

Prevalence

It has been estimated that 20–40 % of elderly hospital inpatients and outpatients have some degree of thiamine deficiency.

Presentation

Acute thiamine deficiency presents as Wernicke's encephalopathy (see also page 138), a delirious state with a classic triad of symptoms:

- Nystagmus

- Ophthalmoplegia (commonly external recti)

- Ataxia.

Other symptoms include ptosis, peripheral neuropathy, pupillary abnormalities, headache, vomiting, confusion, anorexia and fluctuations in consciousness. Untreated it has 20 % mortality, and 75 % will develop Korsakoff's syndrome (page 138).

Treatment

Oral thiamine supplementation is inadequate for treatment. Intravenous or i.m. administration of a multivitamin supplement such as Pabrinex is given.

Vitamin B12 deficiency

Vitamin B12 deficiency is a frequent finding in the elderly. It is an important exacerbating cause of confusion and in a minority of cases a reversible cause of dementia.

Prevalence

It has been estimated that Vitamin B12 deficiency affects 10–15 % of the over 60s.

Aetiology

Only a small percentage of cases of B12 deficiency are due to pernicious anaemia (PA). In the elderly, *malabsorption* and *insufficient diet* are commonly responsible for B12 deficiency.

Presentation

Vitamin B12 deficiency may present with symptoms of fatigue, depression, dementia, weakness, ataxia, peripheral neuropathy and/or subacute combined degeneration of the spinal cord.

Investigation

Patients with a B12 deficiency frequently also have a macrocytic anaemia, but absence of anaemia and/or macrocytosis cannot be taken to indicate normal B12 reserves. Thus serum B12 must be measured in any patient with clinical manifestations that could be due to B12 deficiency.

Treatment

B12 injections are given i.m. daily for five days, and then every three months. Any reversible causes of malabsorption should be investigated and treated as appropriate. It is imperative to ensure there is no folate deficiency before replacing B12.

Neoplastic disease

Systemic neoplasia may result in neurological or psychiatric complications secondary to metastasis, metabolic/endocrine disturbance or stroke. Furthermore, medications given to patients with cancer commonly have neuropsychiatric side effects.

In some cases, however, neurological and psychiatric complications of malignancy cannot be directly attributed to the above causes but to a *paraneoplastic syndrome*. The major subtype of interest to psychiatry (although exceedingly rare) is *paraneoplastic limbic encephalitis* (PLE). The pathogenesis of PLE is autoimmune. PLE can present with seizures, memory problems, irritability, depression, confusion and dementia. It is most commonly associated with small cell lung tumours, testicular cancer and breast cancer.

Presentation

Neuropsychiatric presentation of malignancy depends on the type of cancer and the site of the lesion. Malignancy may cause a variety of symptoms including anxiety, depression, fluctuating or rapidly progressing cognitive impairment over days or weeks, dementia and personality changes.

Treatment

The primary treatment is identification and treatment of the tumour. Any pharmacological treatment for behavioural disturbance secondary to malignancy should take into account the patient's physical state and interactions with other medication.

The psychological impact of terminal illness and its management is outlined in the palliative care section.

Palliative care

Palliative care is a relatively new specialty. This section covers the role of the psychiatrist in palliative care, including pain management, helping the patient with adjustment to their illness, and assessing and treating mood disorder, hallucinations and delusions.

In particular, it is worth noting that end stage dementia is a terminal illness, and that palliative care is therefore a necessary aspect of its management.

Although the WHO definition of palliative care (Box 14.16) precludes physician-assisted suicide, this has nevertheless been legalised in some countries, and the role of the psychiatrist in this controversial area of medicine is outlined in the final section below.

Pain management

Whilst an increasing number of hospitals employ specialist pain teams, it is still possible that cases of treatment-resistant pain may be referred to liaison psychiatrists. Treatment-resistant pain may be a somatisation symptom of anxiety/depression; guidelines for diagnosis and treatment of depression in palliative care are given in the "Mood disorders" subsection below.

Box 14.16   WHO (1990) definition of palliative care

Palliative care:

−affirms life and regards dying as a normal process

−neither hastens nor postpones death

−provides relief from pain and other distressing symptoms

−integrates the psychological and spiritual aspects of patient care

−offers a support system to help patients live as actively as possible until death

−offers a support system to help the family cope during the patient's illness and in their own bereavement

---

Pharmacological treatment

Polypharmacy is common in palliative care, and therefore any new medication should be prescribed with caution.

Low-dose amitriptyline (at a starting dose of 10 mg o.d.) can be useful for neuropathic pain, but side effects from higher doses may be particularly troublesome in palliative care patients (see below).

Psychological treatment

The role of psychological intervention in palliative pain control is controversial. There is limited evidence for the use of CBT and relaxation techniques.

Adjustment disorders

Adjustment disorders are the most common psychiatric presenting complaints in palliative care. Following the diagnosis of an incurable illness, patients may go through the stages of denial, anger, bargaining, depression and acceptance. These states may exist simultaneously and are not necessarily experienced by all.

In particular, palliative care patients may fear:

- Physical disfigurement and pain

- Loss of autonomy

- Financial hardship

- Abandonment by friends and family

- Becoming a burden

- The end of existence

- Loss of control of bodily functions and/or behaviour or mental ability during the final stages of life.

Psychiatric assessment and treatment is indicated if the patient's adjustment is severely impairing their function and/or quality of life, or if there is doubt as to the diagnosis.

Pharmacological treatment

If symptoms are particularly pronounced or prolonged, antidepressant therapy should be considered. See the "Mood disorders" section below for advice on antidepressant treatment in palliative care.

Psychological treatment

Supportive psychotherapy and practical assistance are the cornerstones of treatment for adjustment disorders. Liaison with local religious ministers attached to the hospital may be appropriate in some cases.

Mood disorders

Whilst it is generally agreed that depression is common in palliative care patients, methodologies of studying the phenomenon differ widely such that estimates of prevalence vary between 10 and 60 %. Systematic review has failed to reveal any preferred method of detecting depression.

Depression may be missed in palliative care patients (see Box 14.17). Diagnosis may depend upon a repeated assessment of the patient with particular reference to the cognitive symptoms of depression (e.g. anhedonia) and detailed knowledge of their premorbid personality.

Suicidality

Talk of suicide is common amongst terminally ill patients. However, this does not necessarily reflect depression or even suicidal intent, as it may be a coping mechanism for dealing with a perceived loss of autonomy.

Box 14.17   Why depression is missed in palliative care

Assumption that symptoms are a natural reaction to illness.

Attributing physical symptoms to illness.

Patient's unwillingness to report symptoms.

Doctor's difficulty in asking about symptoms.

Source: Dein (2003)

Suicidal intent may fluctuate with physical symptoms of illness, and so may be amenable to appropriate physical palliative care in addition to psychiatric intervention.

Pharmacological treatment

Box 14.18   Pharmacological treatment of mood disorders in the presence of medical co-morbidity

Assess renal and hepatic function before prescribing.

Check interactions with other medication.

Start antidepressants at a low dose.

Limited evidence to suggests SSRIs have advantages over TCAs in terms of mood and pain intensity.

SSRIs may also be advantageous in terms of interaction with other medications and side-effect profile.

TCAs may help with neuropathic pain, but also have side effects such as constipation, urinary retention, mouth dryness and anticholinergic delirium.

Benzodiazepines may be of use in treating anxiety, but are used with caution in patients with hepatic and respiratory impairment.

Psychological treatment

In the absence of conclusive evidence for the use of psychotherapy in depressed palliative care patients, it is possible that CBT and supportive psychotherapy may be of some benefit.

Hallucinations and delusions

Hallucinations and delusions are common in terminal illness. The delirium chapter of this section covers the assessment and treatment of these acute symptoms in detail.

In addition, many palliative care patients report that they are visited by the "ghosts" of dead relatives and can often have pleasant conversations with them. Intervention with antipsychotic medication is not appropriate if the experience is comforting and does not result in behavioural disturbance.

Physician-assisted suicide

Although it is within the right of any patient with capacity to refuse treatment, assisted suicide is illegal in the vast majority of countries. However, physician-assisted suicide is at the time of writing legal in the Netherlands, Belgium, Switzerland and the US state of Oregon.

Patients requesting assisted suicide may be referred for a psychiatric opinion. It is recommended that such referrals are dealt with by a senior and experienced colleague. A full psychiatric assessment is carried out with specific regard to the questions of whether the patient has capacity to make this decision, and whether this request is consistent with what is known of their premorbid personality. A key aspect of this assessment is to exclude any contribution of depression, psychosis or cognitive impairment.

Further reading

Delirium

Fick D, Agostini J, Inouye S (2002) Delirium superimposed on dementia: a systematic review *J Am Geriat Soc* 50: 1723–1732.
Inouye S (2006) Delirium in older persons *New Engl J Med* 354: 1157–1164.

Epilepsy

Brodie M and Kwan P (2005) Epilepsy in the elderly: clinical review *BMJ* 331: 1317–1322.
Butler C and Zeman A (2005) Neurological syndromes which can be mistaken for psychiatric conditions *J Neurol Neurosur* 76: 31–38.

Parkinson's disease

Chaudhury K, Healy D, Schapira A (2006) Non-motor symptoms of Parkinson's disease: diagnosis and management *Lancet Neurol* 5: 235–245.

CNS infection

Dolder C, Patterson T Jeste D (2004) HIV, psychosis and aging: past, present and future *AIDS* 18: S35–S42.
Hutto B (2001) Syphilis in clinical psychiatry: a review *Psychosomatics* 42: 453–460.

Rheumatological disease

Boddaert J, Huong D, Amoura Z *et al.* (2004) Late-onset systemic lupus erythematosus *Medicine* 83: 348–359.
D'Cruz DP (2006) Systemic lupus erythematosus *BMJ* 332: 890–894.
Savage C, Harper L, Cockwell P, Adu D, Howie A (2000) ABC of arterial and vascular disease: vasculitis *BMJ* 320: 1325–1328.

Neoplastic disease

Voltz R (2002) Paraneoplastic neurological syndromes: an update on diagnosis, pathogenesis, and therapy *Lancet Neurol* 1: 294–305.

Palliative care

Dein S (2003) Psychiatric liaison in palliative care *Adv Psychiat Treat* 9: 241–248.
Hotopf M, Chidgey J, Addington-Hall J, Lan Ly K (2002) Depression in advanced disease: a systematic review. Part 1: prevalence and case finding *Palliative Med* 16: 81–97.
Lan Ly K, Chidgey J, Addington-Hall J, Hotopf M (2002) Depression in advanced disease: a systematic review. Part 2: treatment *Palliative Med* 16: 279–284.
Okie S (2005) Physician-assisted suicide – Oregon and beyond *New Engl J Med* 352: 1627–1630.
Terry W, Olson L, Wilss L, Boulton-Lewis G (2006) Experience of dying: concerns of dying patients and carers *Int Med J* 36: 338–346.

Appendix 1
The Geriatric Depression Scale

A score of one is given for each of the answers indicated in bold type in Box A1.1.

- Score of five or above: possible depression

- Score of ten or above: probable depression

Box A.1   GDS

Choose the best answer for how you have felt over the past week:

1. Are you basically satisfied with your life? YES/**NO**

2. Have you dropped many of your activities and interests? **YES**/NO

3. Do you feel that your life is empty? **YES**/NO

4. Do you often get bored? **YES**/NO

5. Are you in good spirits most of the time? YES/**NO**

6. Are you afraid that something bad is going to happen to you? **YES**/NO

7. Do you feel happy most of the time? YES/**NO**

8. Do you often feel helpless? **YES**/NO

The Old Age Psychiatry Handbook   Joanne Rodda, Niall Boyce, and Zuzana Walker
© 2008 John Wiley & Sons, Ltd

9. Do you prefer to stay at home, rather than going out and doing new things?
YES/NO

10. Do you feel you have more problems with memory than most? **YES**/NO

11. Do you think it is wonderful to be alive now? YES/**NO**

12. Do you feel pretty worthless the way you are now? **YES**/NO

13. Do you feel full of energy? YES/**NO**

14. Do you feel that your situation is hopeless? **YES**/NO

15. Do you think that most people are better off than you are? **YES**/NO

Score = /15

Appendix 2
Testing the function of specific lobes

The dominant lobe is usually the opposite of the hand that the patient writes with.

Frontal lobe testing

Table A2.1 Frontal lobe tests

Motor sequencing	Luria's motor test – demonstrate making a fist, then open your hand out, then rest your hand palm-down. Repeat and check that the patient can copy this sequence, each hand in turn.
Verbal fluency	"How may words can you think of that begin with A? S? F?" Give the patient one minute for each. The combined number of words should be 30 or above.
Category fluency	"How many animals with four legs can you think of?" Allow one minute.
Abstract reasoning	"What would I mean if I said 'a stitch in time saves nine'?" Any proverb will do for this question, but make sure it's one whose meaning is clear to *you*.
Abstract similarities	"In what way are a pear and a banana like each other?" The answer needs to be specific – "You can eat both of them" is *not* correct.
Cognitive estimates	"How many elephants are there in France?" "How tall is a double-decker bus?"

The Old Age Psychiatry Handbook   Joanne Rodda, Niall Boyce, and Zuzana Walker
© 2008 John Wiley & Sons, Ltd

During the physical examination, primitive reflexes can be tested:

Table A2.2   Primitive reflexes (part of frontal lobe testing)

Glabellar tap	Tap the patient gently between the eyebrows. Normally, the patient will stop blinking after a few taps. This response will be impaired in patients with frontal lobe damage or Parkinsonism.
Palmomental reflex	Firmly stroke the thenar eminence. This sign is positive if you observe a contraction of the mentalis muscle (the lips will curve upwards in an inverted "U" shape).
Rooting reflex	Stroke the patient's cheek laterally from the lips outwards. This sign is positive if the patient's mouth moves as if to take the finger in his or her mouth.
Grasp reflex	Ask the patient to lay both hand flat, palms up. Place your fingers on the patient's palm after saying "Do not take my fingers." This sign is positive if the patient grasps your fingers.

Parietal Lobe Testing

Table A2.3   Features and tests of dominant parietal lobe impairment ("Gerstmann's Syndrome")

Dyscalculia	Ask the patient to carry out some simple mental arithmetic.
Agraphia	Ask the patient to make a simple drawing.
Right-left disorientation	"Can you touch your right ear with your left hand, please?"
Finger agnosia	"Can you point to your left ring finger with your right index finger, please?"
Receptive dysphasia	Note during assessment.

Table A2.4   Features and tests of non-dominant parietal lobe impairment

Spatial neglect	Ask the patient to draw a clock face. If one half is incomplete or missing, neglect is present.
Prosopagnosia	Ask about difficulty recognising faces. If you have a newspaper to hand, you can ask the patient to identify a photograph of a well-known face (e.g. the US President).
Anosagnosia	This phenomenon, of the patient failing to recognise a body part disabled by stroke, will generally become obvious during the history.
Constructional apraxia	Ask the patient to copy the intersecting pentagons (see Appendix 3).
Topographical dissociation	Again, this feature, of difficulty orientating oneself spatially and getting lost in new surroundings, will normally come up in the history.

Damage to both lobes will affect:

Table A2.5 Features and tests of bilateral parietal lobe impairment (will occur in addition to those in Tables A2.3 and A2.4)

Agraphagnosia	Ask the patient to close their eyes. Trace letters on the patient's palm, asking him or her to identify them correctly.
Asteroagnosia	Ask the patient to close their eyes. Hand them an everyday object such as a pen and ask them to identify it.

Temporal Lobe Testing

Dominant temporal lobe function can be tested by examining verbal skills and semantic memory.

Table A2.6 Features and tests of dominant temporal lobe impairment

Verbal skills	Ask the patient to repeat individual words, and then to repeat a full sentence. Ask the patient to read a line of text. Ask the patient to write a sentence. Test knowledge of antonyms: "What is the opposite of high?"
Semantic memory	Ask the patient to repeat an address: "Dr MacKay, 42 West Register Street, London". Inform them that you will ask for it again in a few minutes. Describe a famous person and ask the patient to name them. For example, "This man was born in Liverpool. He was one of the world's most famous pop stars. He recorded a song called 'Imagine'. He was killed in 1980" (John Lennon). Ask the patient to tell you about a famous person, e.g. Marilyn Monroe. If time permits you can ask the patient to identify or to give you details of famous landmarks. Finally, ask the patient to recall the address above.

Non-dominant temporal lobe impairment will impair visual skills and memory.

Table A2.7 Features and rests of non-dominant temporal lobe impairment

Visual memory	Ask the patient to draw the intersecting pentagons (as in the MMSE), and to remember them. Test again after a few minutes.
Anomia	Ask the patient to name a wristwatch and a pen.
Prosopagnosia	Test for memory of faces as above.
Hemisomatoagnosia	This phenomenon, when a patient believes that their limb is in fact alien to them, should become clear from the history.

Bilateral temporal lobe impairment is indicated if the history reveals impaired short- and long-term memory loss.

Upper quadrantanopias found on *visual field testing* in the neurological examination will also indicate temporal lobe lesion. For example, a right homonymous upper quadrantanopia indicates a left temporal lobe lesion.

Appendix 3

The MMSE

Table A3.1 The MMSE

Orientation	"What is the year? Season? Month? Date? Day of the week?"	1 point for each.
	"What country? County? Town? Building? Floor?"	1 point for each.
Registration	"Repeat after me: apple, table, penny."	1 point for each item correctly recalled.
	Record number of attempts.	
Now say "I'd like you to remember those, because I'll ask you for them again in a few minutes."		
Attention	"Can you take seven from a hundred? Then seven from the answer?"	Ask to repeat five subtractions of seven. 1 point for each correct subtraction.
	Alternatively:	1 point for each correct letter in the correct sequence.
	"Can you spell 'WORLD' backwards?"	
Recall	"What were those three objects I asked you to remember a few minutes ago?"	1 point for each.
Naming	Ask the patient to name a pen and a watch.	1 point for each.
Repeating	"Please repeat after me: 'No ifs, ands, or buts.'"	1 point.
Three-stage command	"When I hand this piece of paper to you, I'd like you to take it in your left hand, fold it in half, and put it on the floor."	1 point for each correct action.
Reading	"Please read this and do what it says." Show patient the sentence "CLOSE YOUR EYES."	1 point.

The Old Age Psychiatry Handbook   Joanne Rodda, Niall Boyce, and Zuzana Walker
© 2008 John Wiley & Sons, Ltd

Table A3.1 (Continued)

Writing	"Please write a sentence."	1 point for a grammatically correct sentence.
Copying	"Please copy this design."	1 point if all angles, lines, and overlap are correct.

TOTAL	**/30**

Appendix 4

Cytochrome P450 enzymes, substrates and inhibitors

The following list is by no means exhaustive.

Table A4.1 Important examples of substrates, inhibitors and inducers of the cytochrome P450 system enzymes

CYP450 subtype	Substrates	Inhibitors
CYP1A2	TCAs	Fluvoxamine
	Fluvoxamine	Ciprofloxacin
	Clozapine	Clarithromycin
	Olanzapine	Erythromycin
	Haloperidol	Cimetidine
	Chlordiazepoxide	Ketoconazole
	Diazepam	Grapefruit juice
	Caffeine	
	Theophylline	
CYP2C	TCAs	Fluoxetine
	Citalopram	Fluvoxamine
	Diazepam	Paroxetine
	Phenytoin	Sertraline
	Omeprazole	Amiodarone
	Propanolol	Omeprazole
		Fluconazole

The Old Age Psychiatry Handbook   Joanne Rodda, Niall Boyce, and Zuzana Walker
© 2008 John Wiley & Sons, Ltd

Table A4.1   (Continued)

CYP450 subtype	Substrates	Inhibitors
CYP2D6	Fluoxetine Fluvoxamine Trazodone Venlafaxine TCAs Chlorpromazine Haloperidol Risperidone Codeine Some β blockers and anti-arrhythmics	Fluoxetine Fluvoxamine Paroxetine Sertraline Clomipramine Haloperidol Fluphenazine Amiodarone Cimetidine
CYP3A	Citalopram Sertraline Trazodone TCAs Atypical antipsychotics Benzodiazepines Carbamazepine Galantamine Donepezil Azole antifungals	SSRIs (not citalopram) Erythromycin, clarithromycin Metronidazole Azole antifungals Grapefruit juice TCAs Calcium channel blockers

Index

Note: Figures and Tables are indicated by *italic page numbers*, Boxes by **emboldened numbers**

The Old Age Psychiatry Handbook Joanne Rodda, Niall Boyce, and Zuzana Walker
© 2008 John Wiley & Sons, Ltd